Tai Chi

THIS IS A CARLTON BOOK

Text and Design copyright © Carlton Books Limited 1999

This edition published by Carlton Books Limited 1999

A CIP catalogue for this book is available from the British Library.

ISBN 1-85868-916-3

Executive Editor: Tim Dedopulos
Editorial Assistant: Sam Wigand
Art Editor: Tim Brown
Designer: Vladek Szechter
Production: Garry Lewis

Printed in Spain by Gráficas Estella, S.A.

Tai Chi

Erle Montaigue

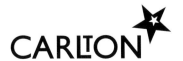

Contents

Introduction

An 'Internal' martial art is one that makes use of the whole body and uses leverage as opposed to brute strength and tension. The Internal arts rely upon a build up of an intrinsic energy or 'Qi' (say, 'chee') to give that something extra in the way of 'internal power'. Over time, we are able to build upon the Qi (energy) that was given to us at birth (pre-natal Qi) to enable us to gain good health and a power that seems to others to be supernatural. However, this internal power is not supernatural, it is quite natural. It allows the mind to use the whole body in total harmony so that when we, for instance, punch, there seems to be much more power manifested than you would find in a 'normal' punch that used only the triceps muscles.

Taijiquan (also known as Tai Chi, T'ai Chi, T'ai Chi ch'uan, Taiji) is considered the 'Mother' of all the 'Internal' martial arts. There are three main internal martial systems from China. Taijiquan is the first of them and its name means, 'Supreme Ultimate Boxing'. Baguazhang (also, Bagua, Bagwa, Bagwazhang, Pa-Kua Chang, Pa Kua) is said to be the 'daughter' or 'sister' of Taijiquan and means 'Eight Diagram Palm'. Its method of fighting and healing is derived from the Chinese 'Book of Changes' or the *I Ching* (say, 'yee jing') which has eight trigrams and 64 hexagrams. Xingyi ch'uan, (also, H'sing-I, H'sing-I ch'uan) the third internal system is considered to be the 'son' or 'brother' of Taijiquan and its name means 'Body-Mind Boxing'.

In China, most internal martial artists practice Taijiquan as their main system plus one other internal system such as Baguazhang. Very rarely will you find someone trying to practice all three! There is an old saying in China which translates as "It would take three lifetimes to learn all three". However, in the West, many people practice all three, and never really master any of them because of it.

Taijiquan is considered to be the pinnacle of Chinese philosophy, healing and self defence. However, not many teachers know how to use Taijiquan for self-defence. Self defence seems to have been lost in a quagmire of mystical mumbo-jumbo somewhere around the late 1960s to the mid 1970s when the 'New Age' movement adopted Taijiquan as its mascot, turning it into a woozy little dance that was supposed to somehow lead to 'enlightenment'.

There are four main styles of Taijiquan, each with further changes or styles introduced within each 'Family' system. I am presenting the Yang Cheng-fu form of Taijiquan in this book. This style was the first to use the all-slow moving form that many people are used to seeing nowadays. It was invented in the mid-1920s by the grandson (Yang Cheng-fu) of the original founder of the Yang Style, Yang Lu-ch'an.

Yang Cheng-fu saw a need for Taijiquan to be taught to all people regardless of age or state of health. He looked at what his father (Yang Chien-hou) had taught him and knew that this more energetic form with leaps and kicks could not be performed by everyone. So he set about changing the style, leaving out all of the *fa-jing* (explosive energy) movements and leaping kicks etc. His form was said to be the most that the original form could be changed without losing the vital essence of Taijiquan. Sadly, others came along and further changed the Original Yang Cheng-fu form, inventing their own 'shortened forms' to the detriment of the art and of people's health.

There are three other sytems. Wu style was finished by Wu Chien-chuan after he learnt Tai Chi it from his father, Wu Quan-yu, who in turn learnt it from Yang Lu-ch'an. The Wu family were Manchu and did not have Chinese surnames, and so were precluded from learning the very famous Yang Family system. Quan-yu used the surname of Wu in order to learn the Yang Tai Chi, and his son refined it into the Wu style.

The Sun style was invented by Sun Luc-tang who was more famous for his Baguazhang than for his Taijiquan. He learnt it indirectly from the Yang Style. He

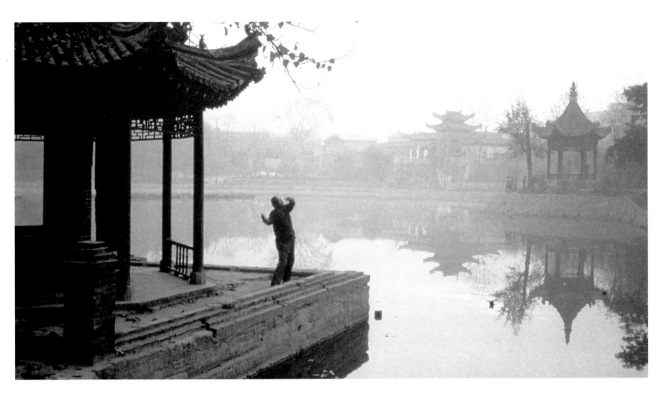

tried to invent a smaller form of Taijiquan that would be performed around the circumference of a circle in the same way as Baguazhang is practised. Sun style Tai Chi is rare nowadays because it didn't quite work.

Finally there is the Chen style. Many people believe that this was the original style, which I dispute.

Within the Yang style, there is some confusion because Yang Cheng-fu changed his Family style four times. He changed it originally so that everyone could practise Tai Chi and gain the great health benefits. The style I present here is Yang Cheng-fu's second version, which is his best system as it incorporates much of the martial aspect as well as the healing side.

The Yang Cheng-fu style of Taijiquan is made up of 37 different postures, many of which are repeated, making a total of 108 which are all linked together by transitional movements. When these postures are performed sequentially we end up with the slow-moving long form. A 'form' is just another name for a set of martial arts movements.

When the long form is performed in this manner it gives us a way of achieving good health, even to the point of healing ailments. It is also one of the greatest self-defence forms ever invented.

The way that Taijiquan heals the body is by balancing the amount of Yin ('negative', female, dark) and Yang ('positive', male, light) energy or Qi within the body. It is said that when a body is in a state of balance regarding Qi, nascent diseases can be healed and those that are developing can be stopped in their tracks. The Chinese believe that all diseases are caused either by an imbalance of Yin and Yang in the body, which allows external pathogens to attack the internal organs, or the body's organs failing to work properly, as in the case of diabetes, etc.. There has been much clinical experimentation done on the healing aspects of Taijiquan in China by respected doctors which provides evidence in favour of the belief in the healing qualities of Taijiquan.

China's history is steeped in the lore of Traditional Chinese Medicine (TCM) so all of the great internal martial systems have this element built in. Balance is the most important area of one's training. I do not mean, however, that we can simply stand on one leg. I mean that all of our six balanced pairs of organs and corresponding body parts are balanced as far as Yin and Yang Qi is concerned. So when the hands, for instance, are balanced with the feet, we will have an equal amount of Yin and Yang energy in these parts.

The six balanced organ pairs with their corresponding acupuncture meridians or acupuncture and *dim-mak* points are as follows:

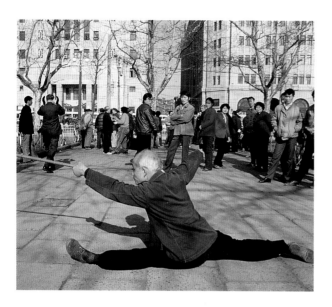

Balanced Body Parts
Corresponding Acupuncture Meridian (Dim Mak)

Hands and **Feet** should be balanced
Stomach & Spleen (ST & SP Meridians)

Knees and **Elbows** should be balanced
Kidneys & Bladder (KD & BL Meridians)

CV1 (Point between the anus and genitals) and **Crown of the Head** should be balanced
Triple Heater Meridian (GV20) & Pericardium meridian (TH & PC Meridians)

Buttocks and **Axilla** should be balanced
Gallbladder & Spleen (GB & SP Meridians)

Coccyx and **Back of the Skull** should be balanced
Heart & Small Intestine (HT & SI Meridians)

Shoulders and **Hips** should be balanced
Lung & Large Intestine or Colon (LU & CO Meridians)

TAIJIQUAN AS SELF DEFENCE

In the martial arts world, Taijiquan is considered to be one of the most effective systems for self-defence. There is a difference between 'martial arts' and 'self-defence'. When Taijiquan was invented, the founders had to have some way of presenting what they had discovered to their own family members and close students without everyone learning their secrets. You must remember that in ancient China a woman would never know if her husband would make it home that evening without being attacked and killed! They taught a dance-like set of movements into which was covertly interwoven the most deadly attacking and defensive methods ever invented. Every move we make in our Taijiquan form has martial application. Even a finger movement can mean a deadly strike to a *dim-mak* (death point) or acupuncture point on the human body.

There are three main disciplines that we learn by practising Taijiquan:

SELF HEALING

This is where we make our own body strong and healthy by balancing the amount of Yin and Yang energy we have. However, there is another area of self-healing. Taijiquan was invented by people of phenomenal insight over many centuries, all of whom knew about the energy (Qi) that flows within the body and how both body and energy were affected by movement. These masters knew about acupuncture and about the 12 main acupuncture meridians (channels) and the 8 extra meridians through which Qi flows, thus bathing every internal organ in life-giving energy.

Qi can also be thought of as electricity. This electricity holds our cells together, a known scientific fact. When we die, the Qi stops flowing and our cells decompose. So the longer we can keep the flow of Qi happening, the longer we live, hence the theory that by practising Taijiquan, we will extend life. Those Taijiquan masters who were not killed in battles, and who neither overindulged in drugs and wine nor ate too much, all lived to a grand old age.

During a day, our Qi flow is 'activated' in a different meridian every two hours. As we have 12 main meridians, this constitutes a 24-hour period. So between the hours of 3 a.m and 5 a.m our 'Lung' meridian is activated by this flow of Qi. Our lungs are our powerhouse, they get us going in the morning after sleep, hence that the lungs are activated by Qi at this time in the morning. Of course, humans now have an unnatural way of sleeping in that we do not go to sleep as the sun sets nor do we rise when the sun rises as the animals do.

Between the hours of 5 a.m. and 7 a.m. the colon or large intestine is activated by Qi hence the common wish to go to the toilet at this time! And so this cycle continues throughout the day with the heart coming into activation between the hours of 11 a.m. and 1 p.m. as this is when we 'animals' are supposed to be the most active.

The old Taijiquan masters knew about this flow and activation from their acupuncture training so they invented the secret set of movements that would emulate this Qi movement. So during the Taijiquan form we cause the Qi to be activated in the 12 main meridians an extra three times during training, one cycle for every third of the form. However, the genius of these masters was such that they were also able to cause the Qi flow and activation to return to where it should have been after practice. So if your training takes 20 minutes, although your Qi has been activated three times throughout the meridians, when you finish, the normal activation cycle is where it should be 20 minutes later.

Every posture was devised so that it worked upon a specific meridian. So when we practice, for instance, the posture called *Brush Knee and Twist Step*, we are healing things to do with the heart. When we perform postures such as *Grasp Swallow's Tail* we are healing things to do with the colon. I have experimented with this group of postures and have given just this set to my students to perform in the morning ten times and each time, by the fifth or sixth run through, they are running off to the toilet!

Every move we make must use Qi or 'electricity' and it is Qi that heals and renews our cells. In order to make any movement, the Qi must be present and flow to the required appendage. For instance, if we wish to close a door, Qi flows to the arm and palm from the Tantien under control of the brain. (The Tantien is an electrical nexus about 3 inches below the navel and inside of the body. This is the place where the Qi is said to be stored ready for action). However, Qi, like blood, must have a pathway along which to pass. Blood has arteries and veins while Qi has 'meridians'. These meridians can reach any part of the body, supplying life-giving Qi to every organ. So when we make a movement, the Qi flows along the correct pathways to get to the portion of the body that is making the movement. Along the way however, it travels through a particular meridian, for instance, the Heart Meridian, thus healing the heart. So we can use movement to cause the Qi not only to flow along the correct pathways, but also to be activated within these pathways.

When I say 'flow', I must clarify this. The Qi that continually flows around the body in a 24-hour period is never stagnant unless there is a problem within the body or organs. Normally it flows in just the same way as blood.

Activation is caused by the meridian automatically increasing in electrical resistance so that a greater EMF (voltage) is produced over the meridian, hence the 'activation'. Note: With electricity, when there is a resistance (such as an appliance) placed across an electrical line, the amount of voltage that is dropped across that resistance is dependent upon the amount of resistance.

So, we have a continual flow. However, there is a holding place for an abundance of Qi that we are able to access at any time. It is called the Tantien (*see above*). So we can also have a 'flow' of Qi from this area to other areas of the body. This flow must pass through the correct pathway in order to do its work. And this is where Taijiquan comes in. The generations of Masters who invented Taijiquan knew about this so they set out to invent a series of movements that would send the Qi through all of the meridians and be activated in those meridians in accordance with the normal activation of Qi in a 24-hour period. They put together a series of postures that they knew would call upon Qi to be sent from the Tantien to all parts of the body and organs via the 12 meridians. So when you practice your Taijiquan form, each posture will be working on a particular meridian and therefore upon a particular organ.

The Postures

If one counts every posture, including the linking postures in the classical Yang Taijiquan form, we see that there are around 300. However, many of these postures are repeated and it is generally accepted that the so-called 'Yang long form' has around 108 postures. But if we only take the very basic postures that have names then that number comes down to 37. Those repeated postures are those that the founders of *H'ao ch'uan* or Taijiquan knew to be very important either for their healing benefits or for their martial applications. Inventors of later, new forms of Yang Taijiquan saw these important postures as being redundant, so they simply changed a great form invented by people of genius and left out these postures, rendering the form almost useless!

HISTORY

In order to understand what Taijiquan is, it is important to know a little of the history of how it was founded as it has changed so much since then. This is by no means a comprehensive history as I have covered this area in other books, and there are so many different theories on the history, that it would take a whole book just to document it all. Therefore, I will concentrate mainly upon the history of my own style's lineage. I will briefly cover the other styles of Wu, Sun and Chen. The following is my version of the history of Taijiquan as I have researched it over the past 30 years. Many, however, believe in their own version of the history. No-one however, can say that he or she knows the definite history of Taijiquan as so little has been left to us.

Many people think that Taijiquan refers to the martial part while Tai Chi refers to the 'mystical' part. This is incorrect, as the name 'Taijiquan' is simply a fuller name for Tai Chi; in the old spelling, T'ai chi is no different to T'ai chi ch'uan.

Meaning literally *Supreme Ultimate Boxing*, ('boxing' is the same Chinese character as 'fist' so *quan* can mean fist too) the name 'Taijiquan' did not come into being until around the later part of the 19th century. It is believed that the name Taijiquan was coined by one of the Wu family of Taijiquan founders. In those days, Taijiquan really deserved its rather lofty name, especially around the time of the man called Yang Lu-ch'an who invented the Yang style of Taijiquan. In fact, it was said that Taijiquan was at its pinnacle when Yang formulated his own system.

In feudal China, the masters, family members and students of Taijiquan did not practise Taijiquan in order to help them perform mudane daily tasks. Nor did they use it to help with lifting things, to have a good day, to help with job interviews, to lose weight, or to be popular at parties. People would learn Taijiquan because it would help save their lives! People needed a means of defending themselves against serious attack. Unlike nowadays when we can call a police officer or buy a gun, they had only themselves to depend upon. Attacks were frequent, and money, possessions and women were all likely to be taken. The violence in the world today is negligible compared to what went on in feudal China. So, how did Taijiquan get to where it is today?

There are a number of different theories as to the beginning of Taijiquan. However, all one has to do is to look at what Taijiquan is when practised at a very advanced level, in order to choose which history you will believe. The history is inextricably linked with performing Taijiquan at an advanced stage. One cannot judge Taijiquan history if one has been only practising for around ten to fifteen years, as a high level of expertise will not have been reached.

One theory is that a man called Chang San-feng saw a fight between a stork and a snake and formulated the whole thing from that! This is rather fanciful and romantic, but not true. There are two separate histories of the invention of Taijiquan . A modern theory is that a family called Chen invented a form of Taijiquan from which came all other forms of Taijiquan. If we look at both the Chen style of Taijiquan and the Yang style, we see that the Yang system could not have come out of the Chen style. They are so different both in physical movement and in internal movement.

The Classics of Taijiquan are very definite as to how we should practise and all one has to do is to follow these lessons left to us by the masters of old. It can easily be seen that the Yang style of Taijiquan has come from no other 'hard'(external) system. It is its own system, whereas it is easy to see that the Chen style has its roots in the Shaolin martial arts. No hard style martial art is like Yang style Taijiquan but one can see many hard styles within the framework of the Chen style.

Many still believe that all the Taijiquan forms came from the Chen style. It is interesting to note however, that not one 'Chen style' master was ever invited to any of the great meetings of Taijiquan masters and styles at the turn of the 20 th century. Several masters have told me that they considered Chen style to not even be Taijiquan. Nowadays, the Chen style is often regarded as one of the great Taijiquan systems across the world. Whether one believes that all Taijiquan came from it or not, it does not take away from the fact that it is a great system of martial art.

Fu Sheng-yuan (the son of the famous Master Fu Zhongwen, nephew of Yang Cheng-fu) has to say about the Chen style and Zhiang Fa in the Chen Village can be found in a handout freely distributed by the son of Fu Zhongwen, where he writes:

" *...one often reads about the four major styles of T'ai chi ch'uan.... Viz.: Chen, Yang, Wu and Sun. However, there is only one Supreme Ultimate Fist that conforms to natural forces and principles.*

"*... It is worthy to note that Chen style is not T'ai chi Ch'uan. Historically Chen Shi has it's origins in Shaolin Ch'uan and was actually known as Pao Choi (Pauchui) or cannon fist. A hard external form does not comply with T'ai Chi Ch'uan principles.... At the time when Yang Lu-ch'an was employed in the household of the Chen master, a great boxer called Zhiang Fa came to the Chen village. Zhiang Fa was the greatest exponent of T'ai Chi Ch'uan of his time. The Chen master was so impressed with Zhiang fa's skills that he invited him to stay and teach T'ai Chi Ch'uan to his household. Thus it was that Zhiang fa taught T'ai Chi to Yang Lu-ch'an...*"

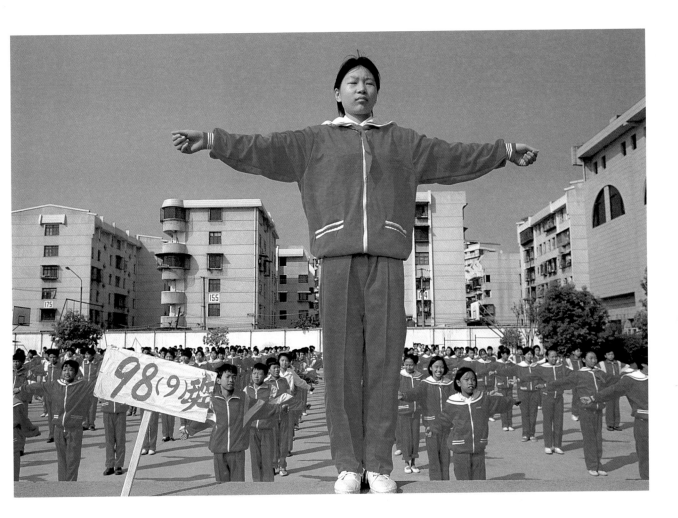

Chang San-feng

It is my belief that Chan San-feng was the founder of Taijiquan, even though the name was not invented back then. One of the main reasons that the Chen family put down the idea of Chang San-feng is that nowhere at the grave of Chang is the word Taijiquan written. There is definitely a Cheng San-feng tomb with many people journeying to this site each year to pay homage. Before the name 'Taijiquan ' it was called *H'ao Ch'uan* or 'Loose Boxing', a name more in keeping with the way that Taijiquan is performed at a high level. Before that, it was simply called *Dim-mak* or 'death point striking'.

Chang was born around 1270 AD. The exact date is open to conjecture, as there are no definite records. So it is only a guess as to when Chang began to invent his system of dim-mak, around 1300.

Chang was a famous acupuncturist in China and

was well versed in the Shaolin system of martial art. He and two other friends were obsessed with the martial arts and wanted to invent the most deadly form of self-defence. They knew from their study of acupuncture that certain points on the human body caused certain electrical and physical effects, so they set about finding out whether these same points could also be used to adversely affect the Qi flow.

The story goes that Chang paid money to the local gaolers to let them experiment on the inmates. Therefore, over a period of trial and error, Chang and his two friends worked out what points would kill, which ones would maim and which ones would affect the Qi (energy) system of the body. They even discovered that certain points would cause great harm or death some time after the strike, hence the 'delayed death touch'. Nowadays, we are able to see why certain points on the human body work the way they do, and indeed, 'delayed death touch' is not just a

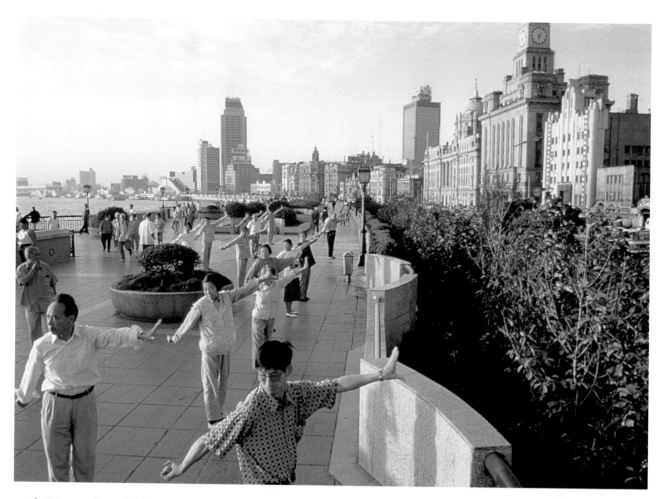

myth, it is actually upheld in modern western medicine.

Everyone in ancient China was looking for the most deadly fighting system so Chang became concerned that others might steal his invention and use it against him and his family. So he had to have a way of teaching it to his family members, a way whereby if someone was looking, they would not be able to work out what was going on. What Chang invented was the very beginning of modern Taijiquan form.

Chang did not just leave it there however; he also wanted to invent a total martial art in keeping with the holistic approach of Traditional Chinese Medicine. So he not only invented physical movements to provide the martial and dim-mak applications, he also invented movements that would heal the body, mind and spirit. He took it one step further in that he had to have a set of movements that could be used to treat others and not only oneself. Hence nowadays we have a totally integrated martial art, one that is used as a deadly self-defence method, a self-healing method and a method of healing physical, mental and spiritual disease in others.

Chang knew that the whole body worked on a combination of brain, muscle, tendon, blood and Qi (electricity). He knew that in order to move anything in the human body, electricity had to be present, and the more electricity (Qi), the more powerful the movement would be. He also knew that in order to cause any part of the body to move, be it a finger or a leg, the Qi had to come from somewhere and go somewhere. The storage place for the Qi is in the kidneys or the Tantien, which roughly corresponds to the point on the *conceptor vessel* (meridian/channel) called CV4. In order for the Qi to go from Tantien to anywhere, it must flow or be *activated* along a sort of electrical conductor. This happens in just the same way that a current will flow over a given path in the electrical mains in your house, for instance. We do not of course have electrical wires running all over the place in our body, but we do have conductors of a liquid type, not unlike the cells of a battery. The current that flows is continually flowing and, if it stopped, we would die. Many people think that the Qi *flows* to certain parts of the body but this is only a more easily understood term that we use to denote *Qi activation* along the meridian. When we need Qi at a certain part of our body, more 'current' is sent along the meridian to the point so that the muscles and tendons will be able to do their work.

This theory is upheld by modern science when one considers that almost all measuring devices in medicine measure voltage or current or magnetic fields caused by those currents. The very cells that we are made of are held together with electricity and when that flow stops, the cells break down and we die. The Qi becomes *activated* along a meridian for two hours for each of the 12 main meridians. It becomes activated by the meridian having a slightly higher resistance at its particular 2-hour period. This causes an increased EMF (electromotive force) or voltage across this resistance hence causing more voltage to create an increase in current along the path. We do not know the mechanism that causes this to happen, but it part of the automatic system of the brain.

So Chang knew that to move an arm, the Qi had to be activated along a certain meridian and through a certain organ thus bathing that organ in life-giving Qi. He set about inventing a set of movements that when executed would emulate the Qi activation cycle throughout the 24 hour period along the 12 main meridians. Not only once – during the whole Taijiquan form, we actually emulate the meridian activation three times. Moreover, even more amazing is the fact that when we finish the Taijiquan form (if it is an original form and done correctly), our Qi activation will be where it should be in the 24 hour cycle. So our energy flow/activation is not put out of whack because we activated each meridian three times in a short period.

Each movement from our Taijiquan form activates the Qi in a different meridian and organ. So when we perform the postures known as *Brush Knee and Twist Step*, in order for the Qi to get to where it should be and to perform that kind of work as denoted by the advanced martial application of the posture, it has to be activated through the Heart meridian. Therefore, this posture will help to heal anything wrong with the heart. In addition, the posture known as *Single Whip*, will heal things wrong with the joints or digestion for the same reason. In fact, every posture from the Taijiquan form will help in the healing of a different organ or disease.

Taijiquan is a series of different postures all linked together as one long slow and explosive moving form. When Taijiquan is performed at an advanced level, there is only one continuous movement from beginning to end.

Wang Tsung-yeuh

Wang was a direct lineage student of Chang San-feng and it is said that Wang was the first of the lineage to write anything down. Before this, the art was passed on by word of mouth for fear that other rival clans would gain this knowledge. As in any family, old letters, notes and bits of paper get stored away somewhere and forgotten. So this treatise became 'lost' for a few centuries until either one of the Chen family, or Yang Lu-ch'an (it is unclear who actually discovered it again) found it lying on either a baker's or a butcher's floor (stories vary).

Zhiang Fa

A man called Zhiang Fa came into the Chen Village at around the same time that Yang Lu-ch'an was living and learning there. Zhiang Fa is said to be a direct student of Chang San-fen via Wang Tsung-yeuh. His fighting style was so good that the Chen family invited him to teach them his system, which he did. He also became friendly with Yang Lu-ch'an and began teaching him. This is all very vague as records are scarce, and the ones we do have cannot be relied upon for accuracy.

The Yang Family

Yang Lu-ch'an (1799-1872) had tried to be accepted into the Chen Village to learn their system, but failed on many occasions. Finally, he acted like a madman, lying in the freezing snow outside the village until someone took pity on him and invited him to live there and become a janitor. It is said that Yang took every opportunity to learn secretly from the Chen even to the point of peeping through holes in doors. Therefore, when Zhiang Fa arrived at the village, Yang was pleased that he was able to learn from him.

Yang became so good at the 'new' system that he eventually left to form his own style called the Yang Style. One story is that Yang also discovered the original treatise written by Wang Tsung-yeuh which helped him to formulate what we now know as the 'Yang Lu-ch'an' style of Taijiquan or the 'Old Yang Style'. This is history is disputed, but it is the version that I find most credible. However, it really doesn't matter what history one

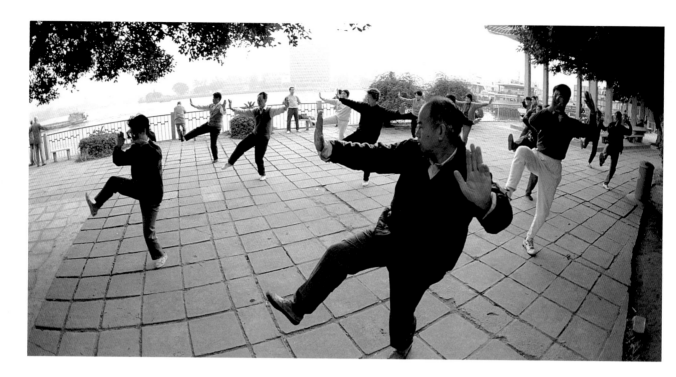

believes as all we have to do is to look at what has been left to us in the form of old writings by the masters and to look at all styles of Taijiquan especially the 'Old Yang Style' and we can easily see that this system is indeed the 'supreme ultimate'. In addition, even if Yang *did* learn everything he knew from the Chen, he certainly improved on that system in the formulation of the Old Yang Style. I call it that because nowadays there are many different systems calling themselves Yang style. However, there is only one true Original Yang Style, that which was founded by Yang Lu-ch'an. Modern Taijiquan owes its invention to Yang's grandson, Yang Cheng-fu but it is very different from the original form.

The Family

Yang Lu-ch'an had six sons and two daughters who were all well versed in the Yang style. The story goes that four of the sons were killed along with Yang Lu-ch'an in a battle with a rival clan. The two remaining sons were Yang Kin-hou (1839-1917) and Yang Ban-hou. (1837-1892). Apparently, Ban-hou went slightly insane at seeing almost his whole family murdered, while Kin-hou joined a Buddhist monastery.

Yang Ban-hou had few students because he was quite brutal in his training while Yang Kin-hou dissemi-

nated the art to his two sons, Yang Cheng-fu (1883-1936) and Yang Shou-hou (1862-1929).

Yang Cheng-fu

Yang Cheng-fu is said to be the modern father of Taijiquan. He changed his father's form three times before he died in 1936. Out of these three changes came three distinct styles of Yang style. We can see these changes in the different versions by Chen Wei-ming, Tung Ying-chieh and Choy Hok-peng, all main students of Cheng-fu and having learnt respectively the different styles as Yang changed the original.

Yang Cheng-fu learnt his father's form as did Yang Shou-hou, but Cheng-fu had an urgent desire to help the Chinese race back to health. So he set about changing his father's form to a more public form, one that everyone, young and old, sick or healthy could gain from. It is said that this form was the most that the original could be changed without losing any of the essence of his father's creation. Others came after Yang Cheng-fu and changed the form even more thus setting the way for the complete destruction of what was once the greatest fighting system ever invented. Nowadays, Taijiquan of the 'Yang system' is no more than a bunch of movements with nothing left of the original internal essence. Being faced with a good karate or street fighter, most modern day 'masters' of Taijiquan would run a mile or be totally defeated in any confrontation. Their excuse for this is that they only teach the 'other side' of Taijiquan, the mystical of healing side. How little they know. We can never take the martial away from the healing, the Yin away from the Yang. When there is Yang in the absence of any Yin or visa-versa, we have nothing! I am afraid that is what most modern Yang style Taijiquan systems are.

Yang Shou-hou

Thankfully, Yang Shou-hou did not change his father's system. He only had, as far as I have been told, three primary students as he was quite brutal in his teaching. One of those was Chang Yiu-chun, who in his older years became my teacher.

Yang Sau-chung

Yang Sau-chung was the eldest of four sons of Yang Cheng-fu. After Yang died, Sau-chung became the leader of the family and in 1949 left for Hong Kong where he lived until his death in 1985 (May). He was born in 1909. I had the pleasure of meeting him in Hong Kong when I went there to train in 1981. He also corrected some of my form via an interpreter. At that time, I was training with Chu King-hung, one of three disciples of Yang Sau-chung, so Chu met me in Hong Kong and introduced me to Yang. Chu wanted me to represent the Yang family in Australasia, and put this to Yang. When I heard the amount that I would have to pay for this privilege, I decided not to play that game and went out on my own. Luckily, I met Chang Yiu-chun.

Qi

The word 'Qi' is not the 'ji' or chi as in the second word in T'ai chi ch'uan or Taijiquan . This 'ch'i' means a 'peak' (ultimate) and its Chinese character looks like a mountain top. Qi as in the internal arts means 'breath' or 'energy'.

Qi, without which we would all die, is the most important aspect of one's Taijiquan training. Qi is given to us at birth and is our life force, the very thing that holds our molecules together. Now it stands to reason that if we have too little of this force then we are not healthy, or if the flow of Qi is impeded, the same result occurs. Therefore, we first have to build up some of this vital stuff so that our internal organs are literally bathed

in the life-giving Qi. However, if we then wish to use this stuff to heal others then we must turn it into a useable form called *jing*.

Jing can be likened to Qi as steam is to water. We gain much 'water' from our Taijiquan and Qigong practise and then we turn it into 'steam' so that we are able to make it work for us. In any given day, our Qi flows around our body twice through the twelve main, and eight extra meridians or channels. These are like electrical conductors that travel around the main organs in the body. During our Taijiquan practise we cause this flow to increase to three extra times around the body for each set or form that we perform.

Every Taijiquan posture causes the Qi to flow through its corresponding organ and so the whole Taijiquan form is made up of these postures perfectly positioned to cause this flow. The reason that this healing art was based upon the 'wushu' or war arts is because the history of China is steeped in war and their whole culture is based upon pugilism. I suppose if Taijiquan were invented in the USA, we would have movements like basketball, baseball or football to follow to give us the appropriate flow of Qi.

Each posture represents a certain martial defensive or attacking movement. This enables us to visualise the actual martial movement which leads the Qi from the *tantien* to the appropriate attacking portion of one's body. Because of the nature of the movements, the Qi is forced to flow through the main organs in order to perform this work and so we have a healing art from a war art.

For those who wish to take Taijiquan on to its secondary stage of a self-defence art — and it is an extremely good one — there are other exercises and forms, faster and more explosive, which teach us this aspect.

Taijiquan is a moving Qigong, or 'internal work'. There are two thousand different types of Qigong broken into three main areas. The most advanced area, and one's final goal in Taijiquan, is to be able to heal others using accumulated Qi in the form of jing. First we must gain some extra Qi ourselves, and to do this we use the basic Qigong stance.

Qigong involves standing in certain postures using various breathing techniques. Much good information about exists, and is available in good bookshops. Using this method, we are able to build upon our 'given' or 'prenatal' Qi. This additional Qi can then be incorporated into the body, and we can draw upon it, and make it flow using the Taijiquan form.

The
Long Form

The Classical Times For Practise Were:

Dawn: When you are coming out of yin and entering yang.
Midday: When you are in extreme yang.
Dusk: When you are coming out of yang and entering yin.
Midnight: When you are in extreme yin.
These times give you a completely balanced practise structure, but most of us can only manage dawn and dusk. True taijiquan is subconscious, where the body and mind are in a state of alpha awareness, not asleep and not awake. Allow your brain to do all the work for you and you can achieve anything. It takes many years to achieve a high level of taijiquan expertise but on the way you will come across many wondrous things and lessons within your life.

Photo No. 1 shows the basic 3-circle Qigong stance to be used when accumulating Qi.

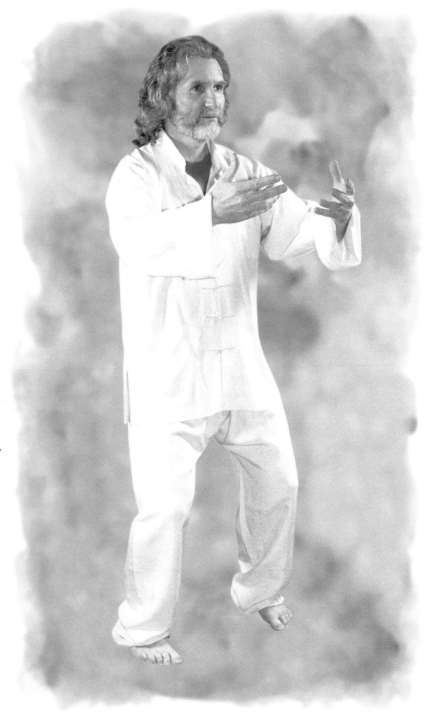

PICTURE 1

YANG CHENG-FU FORM: PRACTICAL

PREPARATION

Stand with feet parallel and shoulder width apart. The palms are at your sides and slightly flexed, but not enough to create tension. This is called a `yang' palm. When the palm is totally relaxed it is called a`yin' palm. The elbows should be held slightly out from the body as if holding a tennis ball under each arm. The energy is sunk to the Tantien. This is the beginning posture. (Photo No. 2). You call the direction that you start off facing 'the North'. This has no real significance other than simply knowing where you are to face. In other words, it does not relate to the Earth's magnetic field.

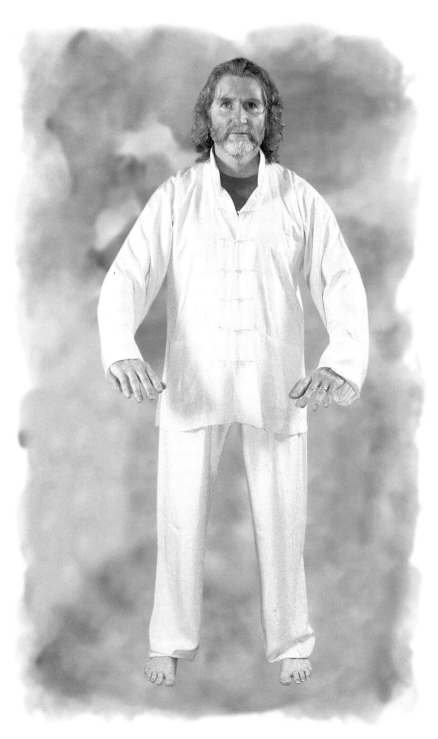

PICTURE 2

Raise Arms

Slowly and deliberately raise your arms up in front of you as if a rope is pulling both palms upward and out from your body. The wrists relax and become yin as you breathe in. The arms are held as if you are sleep walking. The palms are about 6″ apart. Do not bend the elbows any more than they were for the beginning. (Photo No. 3). As you breathe out, slowly and at the same pace, bring the wrists to below the fingers (rather than flexing the fingers upward) and bring the arms back down in the same arc. There can be a slight bringing of the wrists inward but do not make a large circle. Do not bend your knees at this point. Your palms end up where they started. (Photo No. 2).
Important Point: When raising the arms and changing the state of the wrists from yang to yin and then from yin to yang, do not just change the shape of your palm to yin then lift your arms. Be sure that the wrists slowly change state over the whole stroke of the movement up then down. A yin shaped hand is one that is 'limp' while a yang shaped hand is one that is flexed. A yin-shaped hand is full of yang Qi while a yang-shaped hand is one that is full of yin Qi.

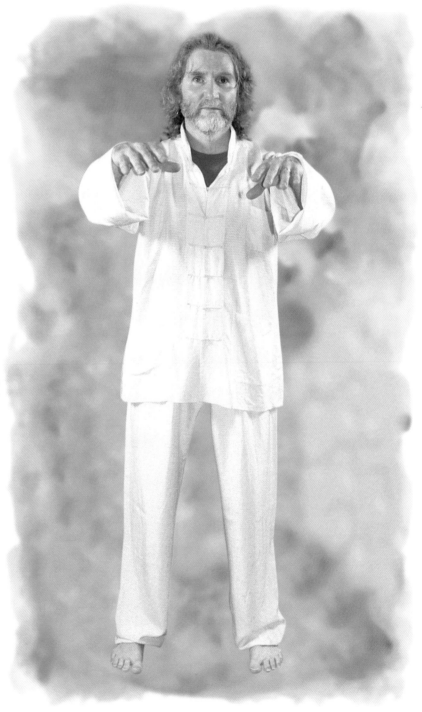

PICTURE 3

20

Push left

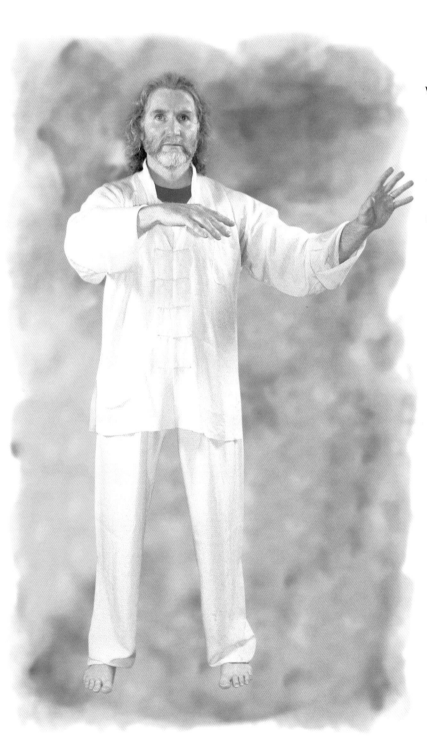

Once again, slowly change the wrists to yin and as you breathe in bring both arms across your body to your right corner, the N.E., in an arc. The palms stay the same distance apart. Keep the left wrist in your centre and away from your body. Inhale. Continue the circle back over to your left, N.W., corner about face height and as your left palm starts to come down, flex the wrist and breathe out. The right wrist is relaxed and in your centre. The left fingers are no higher than shoulder height and the 'Colon 4' points are in line. Exhale. ('Colon 4' points are located in the muscle between the thumb and forefinger on the back of your hand). (Photo No. 4).

PICTURE 4

Block to the right

On that last out-breath bring your left palm down and across your body to end up underneath your right palm. As you do this you should bend the knees placing 70% of the weight onto the left leg. Your right toe swivels to point to the N.E. corner. Your eyes are still on the North but the body has turned. (Photo No. 5). Inhale. *N.B: Unless otherwise stated your weight is always distributed 70% on one leg and 30% on the other.*

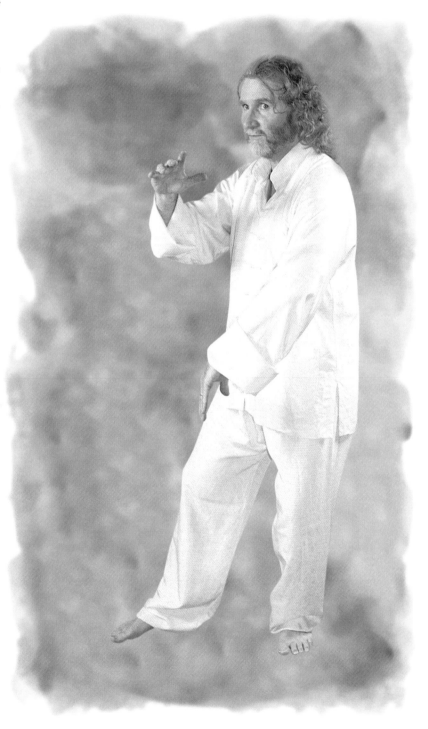

PICTURE 5

P'eng

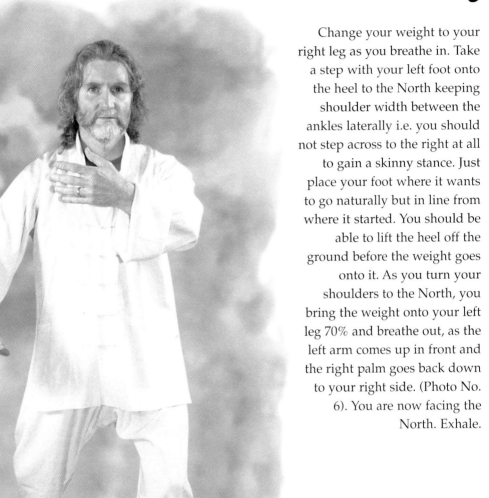

Change your weight to your right leg as you breathe in. Take a step with your left foot onto the heel to the North keeping shoulder width between the ankles laterally i.e. you should not step across to the right at all to gain a skinny stance. Just place your foot where it wants to go naturally but in line from where it started. You should be able to lift the heel off the ground before the weight goes onto it. As you turn your shoulders to the North, you bring the weight onto your left leg 70% and breathe out, as the left arm comes up in front and the right palm goes back down to your right side. (Photo No. 6). You are now facing the North. Exhale.

PICTURE 6

Block to the left

Three movements happen simultaneously. Relax the right palm and bring it under the left. The left palm has turned down to meet it. Pick up the right heel and look to the right (E). Turn your torso to the N.E. and breathe in. (Photo No. 7). Inhale.

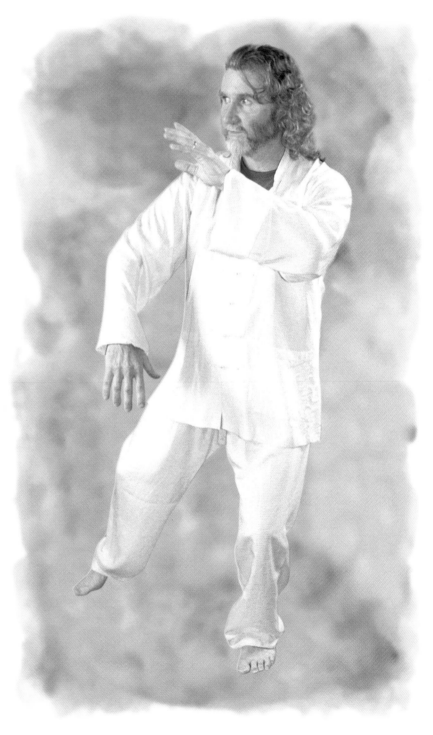

PICTURE 7

Double P'eng

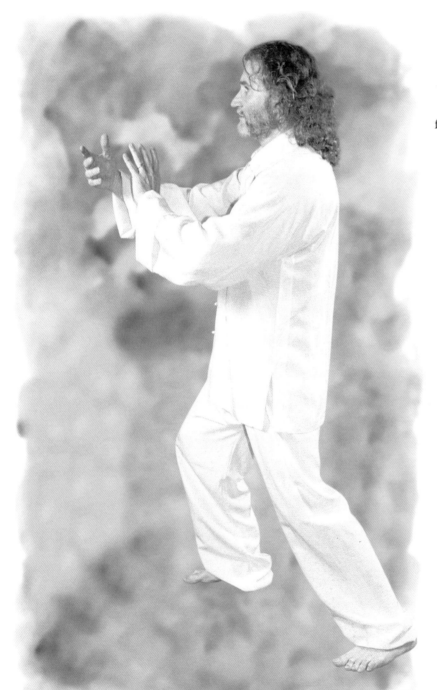

Pick up your right foot and place the heel down almost in the same spot but with the toes facing East. Roll onto the right foot as the right palm comes up in front of your left palm, which does not move but only flexes. The two palms are as if you are holding a small ball between them. You are now facing the East, and your left toes are dragged around by 45 degrees to face the N.E. 70% of your weight is now on your right leg. Breathe out. (Photo No.8).

Lu, or pull back

Turn both palms over (no breath) so that the right is down and the left is facing up. The fingers of the left hand should point into the thumb of the right hand. Both palms pull down to your left hip as your body turns to your left to the N.E. Breathe in. Weight on your left leg. Inhale. (Photo No. 9). *NB: You must turn your body in order for the hands to move to the corner. Do not simply move your arms. The arms only move up or down with the body causing the lateral movement by the movement of the waist.*

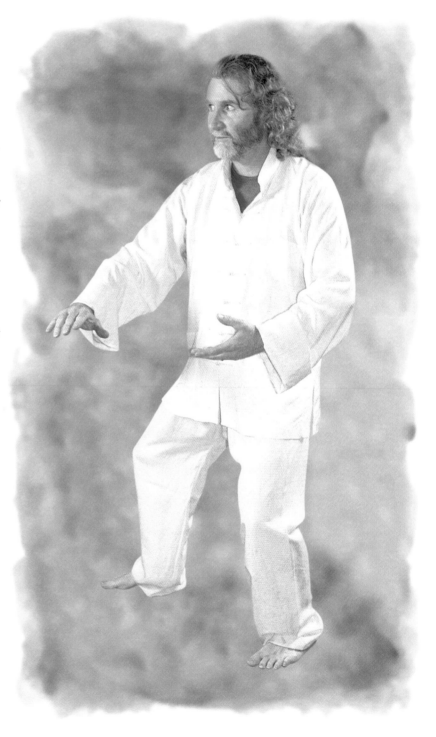

PICTURE 9

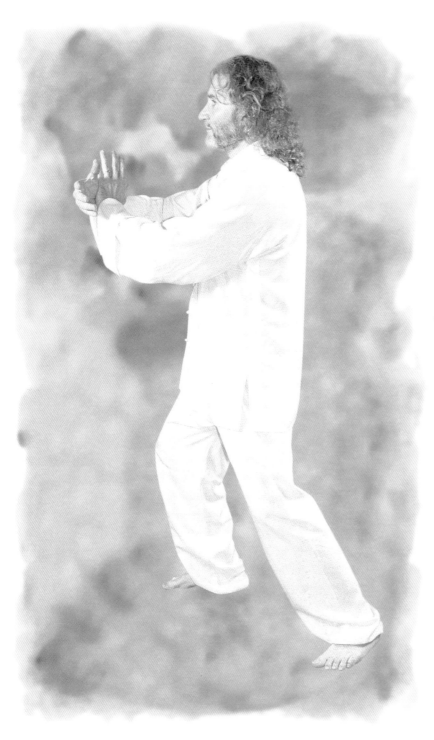

Chee, or squeeze forward

This posture is sometimes wrongly called `press'. This has come from an early mistranslation of the Chinese word. Place the heel of the left palm onto the inside of the right wrist which turns over to face you. Don't lift your palms up and then lift forward but rather bring both palms up in an arc back up to the East as you slightly squeeze your elbows inward and turn back to the East. Breathe out. (Photo No. 10).

NB: When you place your left palm onto the radius of your right arm near the wrist, be sure that it is in a 'yin' shape and that the right palm maintains its 'yang' shape until you execute this strike, only then will both palms release their respective energies and change shape physically.

Sit Back Ready

Brush the top of your right palm with your left palm and extend your fingers palms downward. Sit back onto your left leg as both palms fold in toward your body as you breathe in. Keep the back vertical. (Photo No. 11).

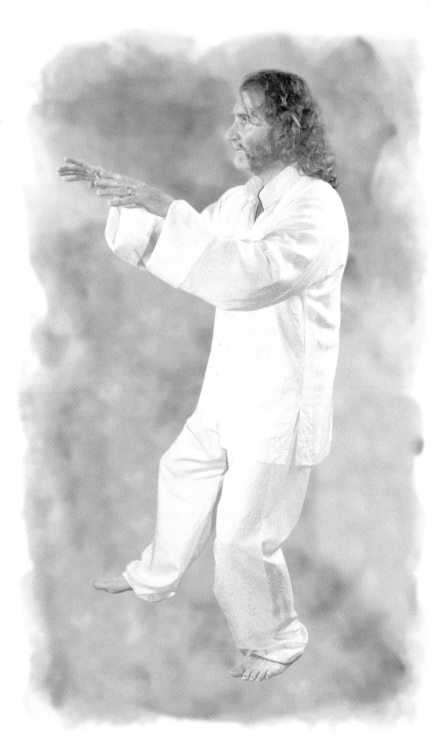

Press forward

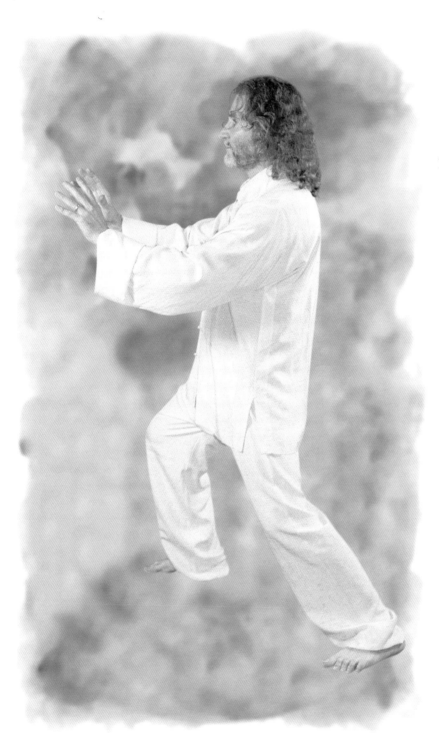

Some people wrongly call this posture push. This has come form an early mis-translation from the Chinese word. From the previous posture, lower your stance slightly and as you flex both palms exhale as you press your palms forward and move onto your right leg. (Photo No. 12). Exhale. With any palm movement, imagine that you are breathing out of your palms from your tantien. *NB: Turn your hips to the East. Do not allow them to relax as this posture should create some small amount of tension in the right inner thigh. Keep your buttocks tucked under and do not allow them to stick out and alleviate the tension.*

PICTURE 12

Sit back ready

Sit back onto your rear foot as you breathe in. Drop the right wrist back to the same position that it was in for photo No. 11, while the other palm, in the same configuration, lies across your chest with the fingers pointing into your right elbow. (Photo No. 13). You are still facing the East. Inhale.

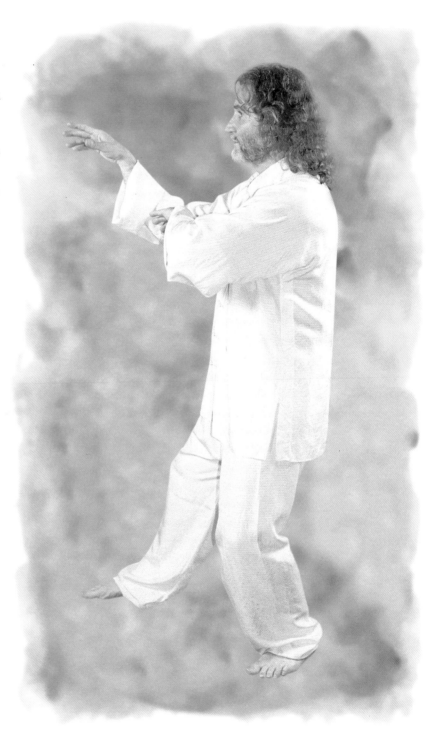

PICTURE 13

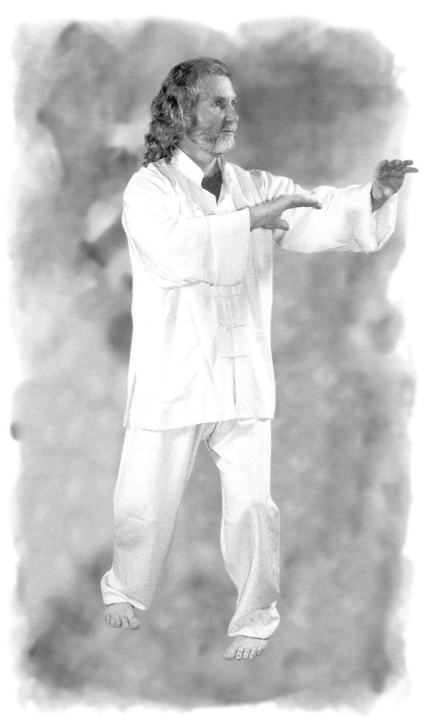

Fishes in eight

With the weight on your left leg, swing both palms out to the left with the left palm leading and both palms flexed away from the movement as if the wind is blowing the fingers backward. The right foot swivels around on the heel by 90 degrees to face North. The left foot is still facing North east. As your left palm and body come around to point North west your right palm comes over to point into your left elbow. This is part of your out-breath. (Photo No. 14). The next half of this movement uses the rest of this out-breath. Bring both palms in towards your chest keeping the palms the same distance apart as you slowly start to change your weight. Turn your body into the N.E. corner with the weight now on the right foot. The position of the feet has not changed. This posture is the exact opposite of Photo No. 14. You have now performed a counter-clockwise lateral circle with both palms.

Single whip

Make a hook with your right palm, all the fingers surrounding the thumb and pointing downwards. The right arm straightens out and points into the N.E. corner. This is the only time that a straight arm is used in Taijiquan. Your left palm turns in to you and the fingers touch the inside of your right elbow as if you are holding a ball in your chest. You should breathe in. Lift up your left foot and leaving the right arm where it is, turn your whole body around taking your left arm with you in the same configuration with left wrist in your centre. Place your left heel down to the west, so that there is shoulder distance between your heels laterally and the foot is to the West as far as it will go without over stepping. The breath has been naturally held. Just before the right heel touches the ground, you should lift your left elbow and do a small inward turning circle and push to the west as your weight comes down onto the left leg. Your right toes are dragged around to point to the N.W. at the last. Breathe out. (Photo No.15).

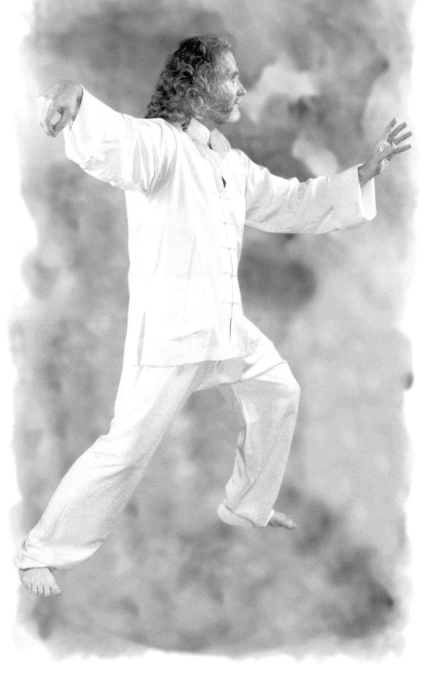

PICTURE 15

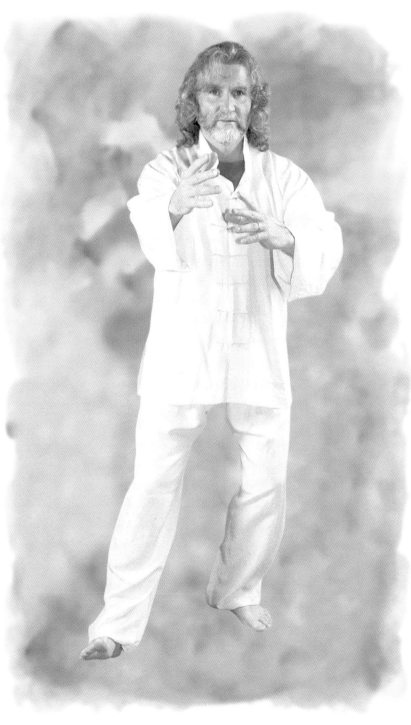

Lift hands

Allow both palms to flex slightly as they are moved down about 6″, as if the arms are wings. Now, on the in breath, lift both palms up again about 6″ and turn your left toes 45 degrees to point to the N.W. This is a heel weighted turn. Flex both hands downwards again and bring them down in two arcs to the front of your body. The left palm is pointing to your right elbow. Lift both palms up as if splashing water onto your face, still with the left palm near your right elbow. As the palms come up you should lift up your right foot. This is all happening on the out breath. As your palms lower into position, your right heel touches the ground with no weight placed on it. (Photo No. 16).
The distance for the `heel stance' is half shoulder width between the heels.

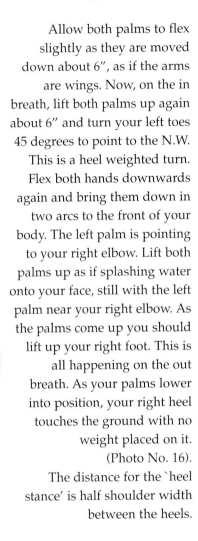

PICTURE **16**

Pull down

From the last position, push both palms out slightly in a down and upward small circle and place a small amount of weight onto the right heel, only about 10%. Turn both palms over, right down and left up, and breathing in pull down to your left side as your body turns to the N.W.
(Photo No. 17).

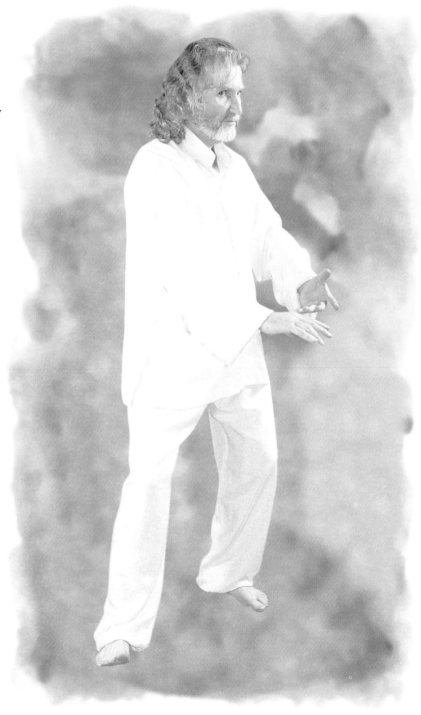

PICTURE 17

Shoulder press

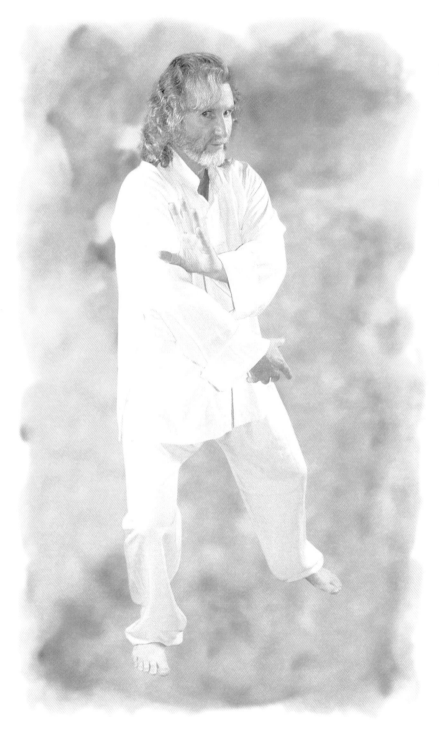

From the last posture, take the left palm in a natural circle and place it onto your right triceps. As this happens, the right foot takes a small step to the N.E. with the toes pointing to the North. This is to make your step larger for the `bow stance', which is shoulder width laterally when dragged back equally. Your body is still turned to the N.W. Now, in posture, you push onto your right foot and attack with your shoulder as you breathe out. Your shoulder should be over your right knee and your back should be vertical (Photo No. 18). At this point your eyes are looking to the North but your head is in its correct position and faces the same direction as the body.

PICTURE 18

Stork spreads wings

Turn your body only slightly to the right as your right arm comes up with the wrist in your centre and palm facing you. Your left palm comes down to your left side. The right palm comes up to chest height and this is part of your last out-breath. Continue the circle of the right palm until it comes over your head and turn to your left, to the West. Your left foot lifts up and is placed down in a `toe stance' with only the ball of the foot touching, but no weight is placed onto it. As you drop into the west, your right palm turns over in a sort of salute. As your palm came up over your head, this was an in breath and as it turned over, this was the out breath. (Photo No. 19).

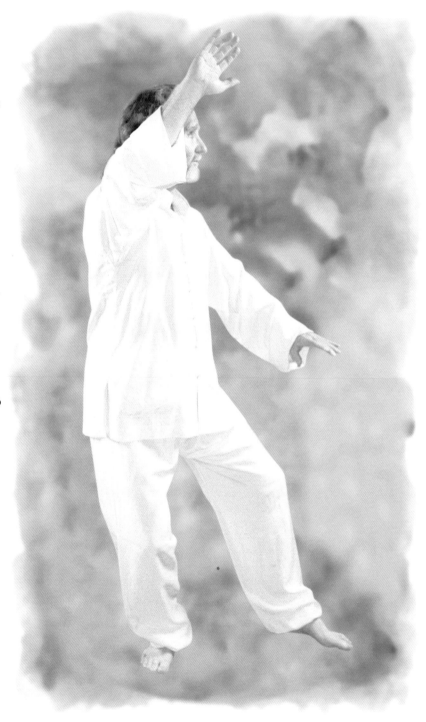

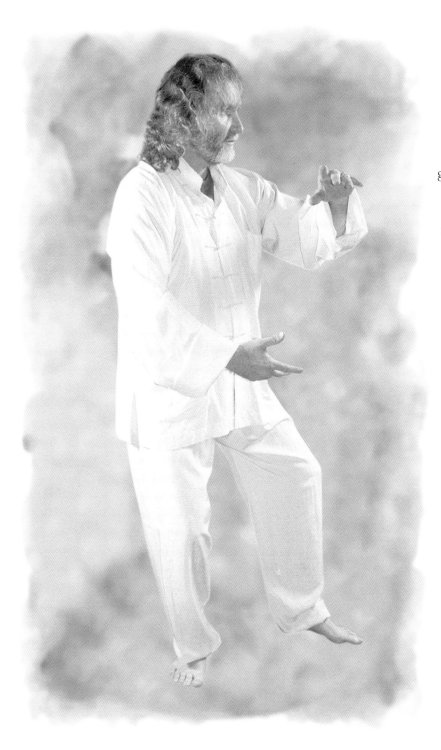

Brush knee and twist step

Drop your right palm down to your right hip and as it moves, you should turn it over palm up. Don't allow your palm to go out to the side in a clockwise arc, just cascade it down. As this happens the left palm relaxes and lifts up to on top of the right palm as if holding a large ball. Breathe in. (Photo No. 20). Your body has turned to the N.W. The left palm continues that same clockwise circle to come down across your body, and the thumb touches your left knee which has lifted to meet it in order to step forward. As this happens, your right palm has lifted up and out to come to ear height.The right palm should not go back from its down position; it should start coming forward with fingers relaxed ready to strike to the West. The breath at this point is naturally held ready for the out breath.

PICTURE 20

Brush knee and twist step

After you have brushed your left knee, your left heel steps to the S.W. with the toes pointing to the West, to gain a bow stance. As the weight is rolled onto your left foot the right palm should come to the West with the body and at the last should flex as the weight comes down onto the left foot. The rear toes are dragged around by 45 degrees to face the N.W. The right index finger is under the nose and you breathe out. (Photo No. 21). This is the difference between a push and a strike. The push starts out with palm already flexed while the strike uses the `flicking up and driving in' of the wrist to strike.

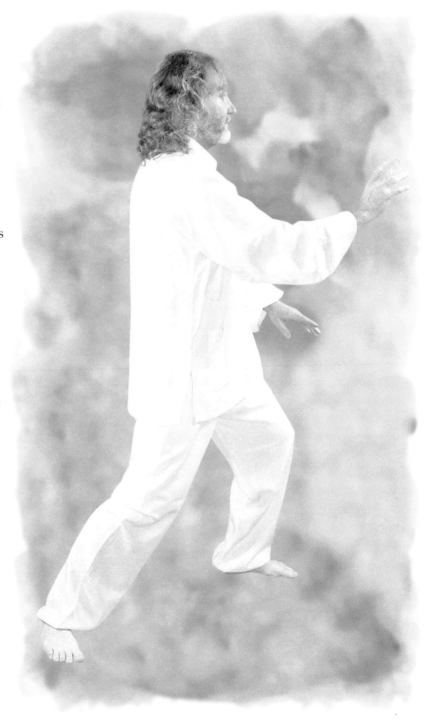

PICTURE 21

Strum the lute

Lift your right foot off the ground about 6″ and place it exactly where it was. Some teachers prefer to bring the foot forward at this point to make it easier but is not correct as it loses its martial value. The lifting of the foot is to cause the left leg to become totally `yang' and so it has maximum thrust backwards. Lift the palms into position as the left heel comes across slightly to form a `heel stance'. As the palms lifted, this was an in breath, and as they dropped into position this was an out breath. This is the opposite posture for `lift hands' but both postures have different applications. (Photo No. 22).

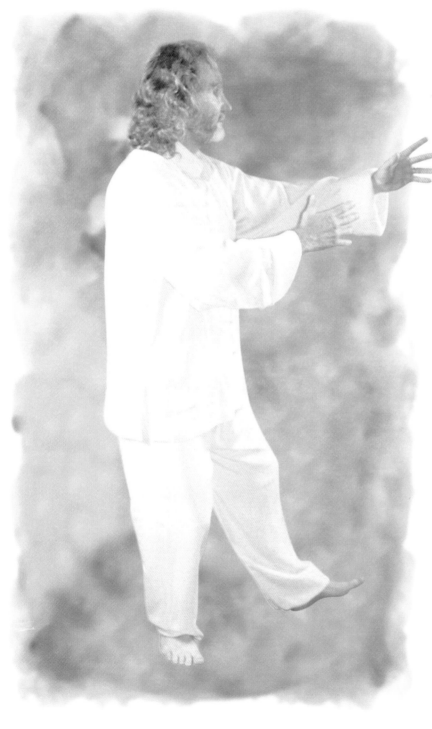

PICTURE **22**

39

Brush knee twist step

Drop the right palm and bring the left palm over to your right corner to hold the ball as you breathe in. Now repeat `brush knee twist step' exactly as you have just performed it. You do not have to drag the right toe around, because it was placed down facing the N.W. (Photo No. 21). This is your second brush knee step. Again perform `brush knee twist step' only this time it is reversed. Turn the left toes 45 degrees to the S.W. weighted, and hold a ball to your left corner, right palm on the top as you breathe in. When you turn your toes out to the corner, do not shift your weight back. As you step to the West with your right foot, the right palm comes down and brushes the right knee as your left palm comes up to your left ear. Place the right foot down to the West and as you roll onto it, strike with your left palm as before. You should breathe out. (Photo No. 23). This is the third `brush knee twist step'.

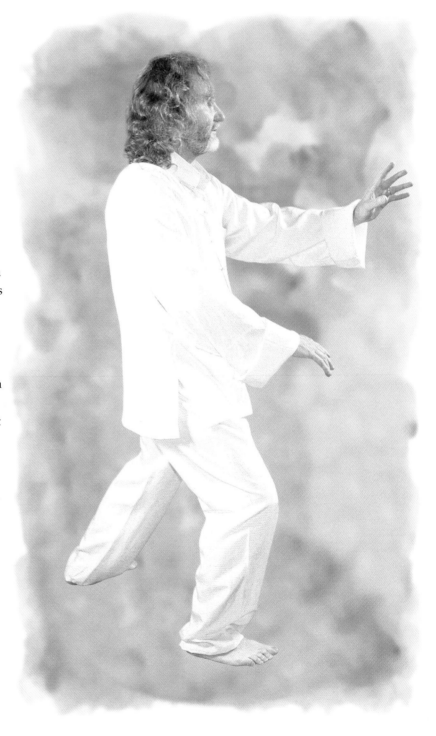

PICTURE 23

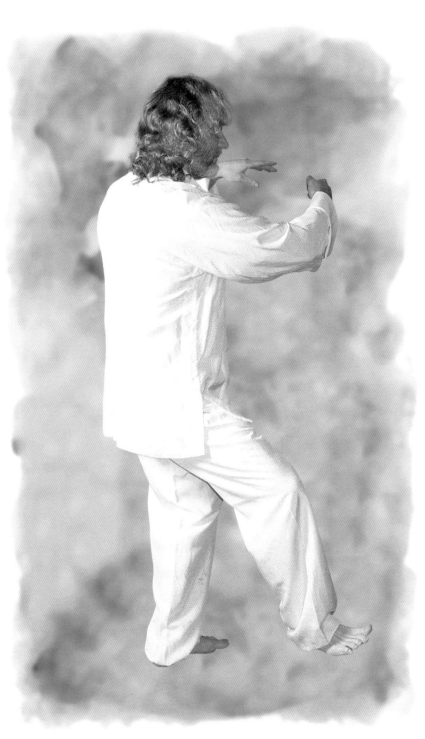

Brush knee twist step

(LEFT FOOT)

A fourth brush knee step. Exactly the opposite to the last posture, turn your right toes to the N.W. weighted on your heel and hold the ball as you breathe in (Photo No. 24). Now brush the left knee as it steps to the West and attack with your right palm. (Photo No. 21).

Strum the lute

Repeat exactly as you did for Photo No. 22.

Brush knee twist step

(RIGHT FOOT)

Repeat so as to finish as in photo No. 21. This is your fifth `brush knee twist step'. So, you have performed one `brush knee twist step' followed by `strum the lute'. Then three `brush knee twist steps' in a row, followed by `play guitar' then another `brush knee twist step' attacking with the right palm.

PICTURE 24

Step forward, parry and punch

With the weight on your left foot, you turn your left toes 45 degrees to face S.W. At the same time the right palm makes a fist and turns palm down. The left palm turns over to face upward at this point. Breathe in. Take your right fist down across to the left side of your body in an arc so that the fingers of the left palm are now pointing into the hole that your right fist makes. Now both palms lift up to ear height, the left palm has turned over to palm down and the right foot has picked up ready to take a step to the West. Block downward with the back of your right arm, palm up still holding a fist, and step to the West with the toes of the right foot pointing N.W. Bring your right fist in to your right hip and as the weight changes to your right leg you should exhale and strike with your left palm. (Photo No. 25).

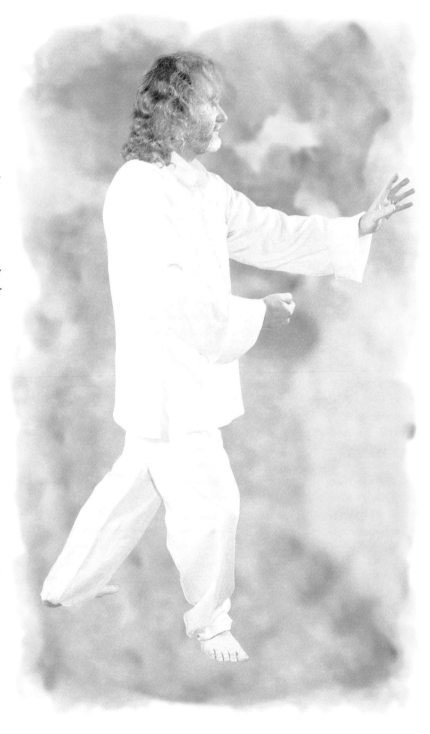

PICTURE 25

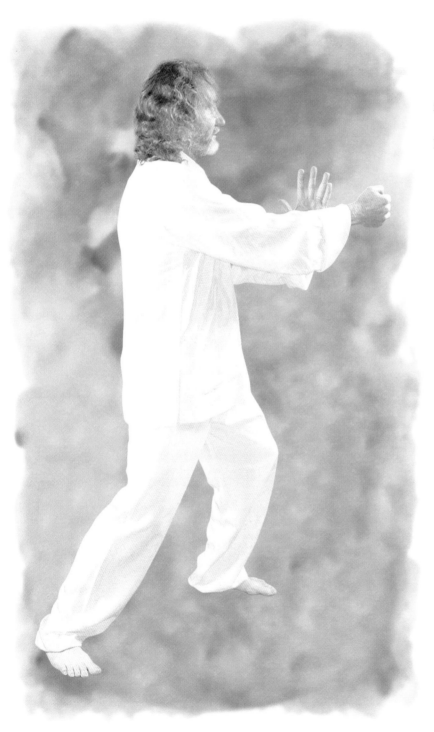

Step forward, parry and punch

Now take a step with your left foot to the West and breathe in. As the weight moves on to the left foot exhale and punch with your right fist to the West. You are now in a left `bow' stance. Your left palm has come back to the inside of your right forearm. The knuckles of the right fist and the tips of your left fingers should be in your centre. (Photo No. 26).

PICTURE 26

Sit back and press forward

Take your left palm and slide it under your right forearm. At the same time, the right palm turns up. The left palm is down. The right elbow is on the left wrist. Leave your left arm where it is and sit back onto your right leg. This will drag your right palm back to your right hip as the left palm turns over to palm up. This turning should happen before your palm reaches the level of your right wrist. Inhale. (Photo No. 27).

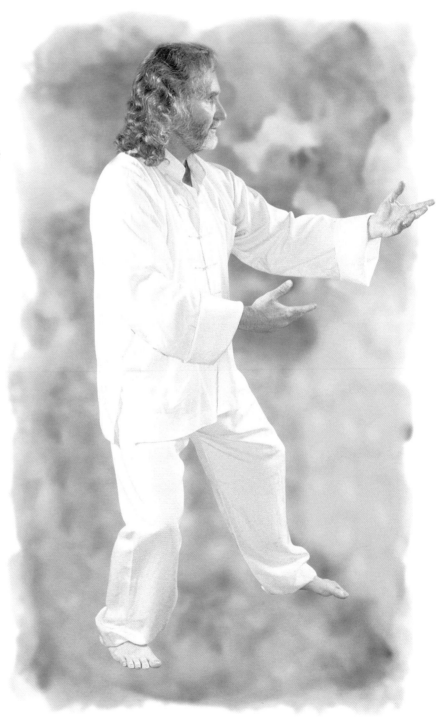

PICTURE 27

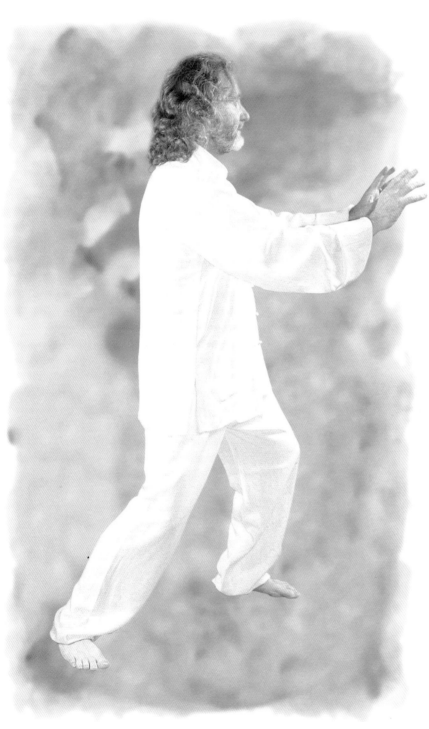

Sit back and press forward

Your body is turned slightly to the N.W. Circle the right palm up so that it is equal to the left palm which has turned out away from you as your torso turns back to face West. Now push forward and squeeze your elbows in slightly as you come back onto your left foot. Breathe out. (Photo No. 28).

PICTURE 28

45

Apparent close up

Holding the palms as they are, lift your elbows slightly as you sit back onto your right leg and Inhale. Turn your left toes 90 degrees to the North, and turn the whole body to face North. Change the weight back to the left leg and open both palms to make two large circles in front of you. The right palm makes a clockwise circle while the left makes a counter clockwise circle. As this is happening the right foot is dragged back to parallel to the left foot and as your arms cross in front of your chest, you change your weight to your right leg. (Photo No. 29). Breathe out. **This is the end of the first third**. *NB: We do not measure the 'thirds' of the form by their amount of postures nor the length of the form. We measure by what the Qi is doing. So when the Qi is settled back to its holding point in the backbone ready for action again after having completed one complete revolution through all 12 main meridians, that is one third.*

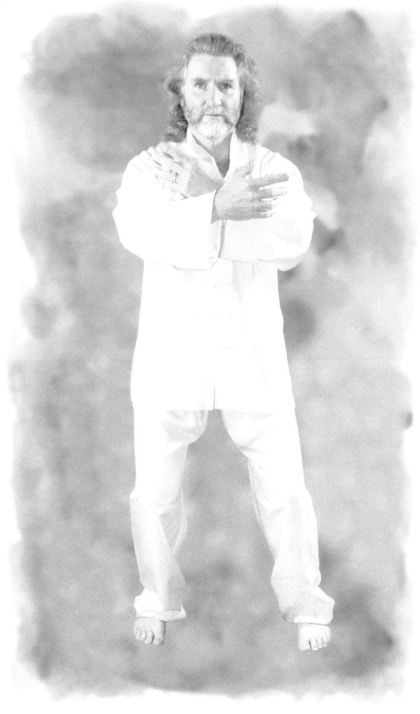

PICTURE 29

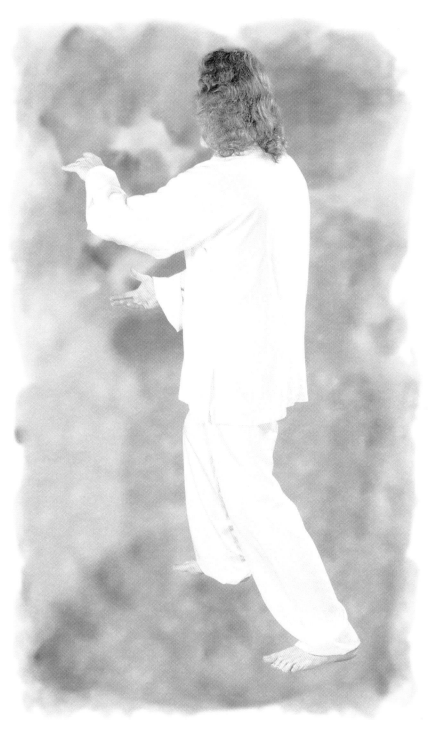

Embrace tiger return to mountain

With your weight still on your right foot, turn your left toes to the right by 45 degrees to point to N.E. Drop your weight onto your left leg as your left palm drops under your right to hold a large ball. Inhale. Now perform `brush knee twist step' in exactly the same way as you did earlier for the right foot forward version. The only difference is that your right foot steps right around into the S.E. corner. You brush the right knee with your right palm and the weight is now on your right leg. Exhale. (Photo No. 30).

PICTURE 30

Grasping swallow's tail

This section duplicates some of the postures done in the first third. Firstly, raise your right palm up to in front of your left palm and Inhale. (Photo No. 31).

Pull back

This is the same as in the first third (Photo No. 9). Turn both palms over, right palm down and left palm up and pull back to your left side as before. The only difference is that you are now facing to the South East instead of to the East.

Chee

This is the same as in the first third, photo No. 10, to the S.E.

Sit back

This is the same as in the first third. (Photo No. 11).

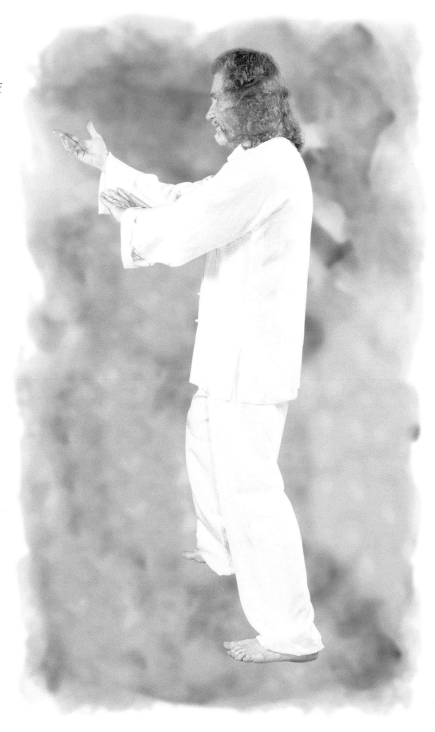

PICTURE 31

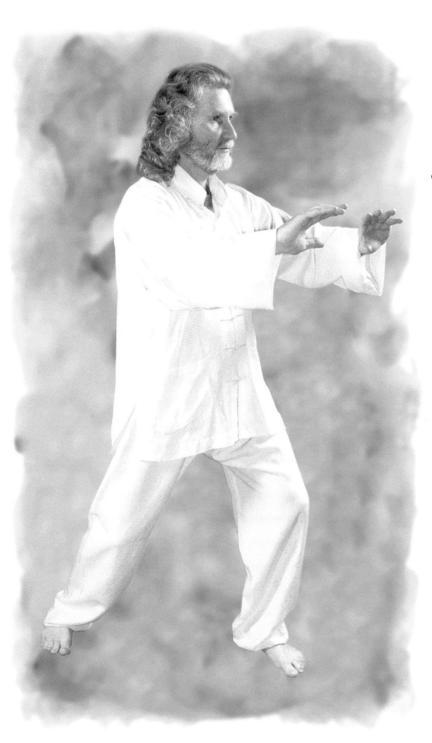

Press to the Northwest

Holding the palms in the `fishes in eight' configuration, you now take a step with your left foot around into the N.W. corner while inhaling. Roll onto your left foot and bring the left palm, which was pointing in to the right elbow, up to equal with the right palm to perform a pushing movement into the N.W. corner. The back toes come around 45 degrees to point to the North. Exhale. (Photo No. 32).

Fist under elbow

Bring your right foot up to equal and parallel to your left foot. You should now be standing on a South West to North East diagonal and facing to the North West with the weight on your left foot. Inhale. As you change your weight to your left leg, cut your right fist in a shallow arc to under your left elbow so that the funny bone sits in the aperture made by the fist. At the same time you should turn your body to the West and make a left heel stance as you exhale. The left index finger is under your nose. (Photo No. 33).

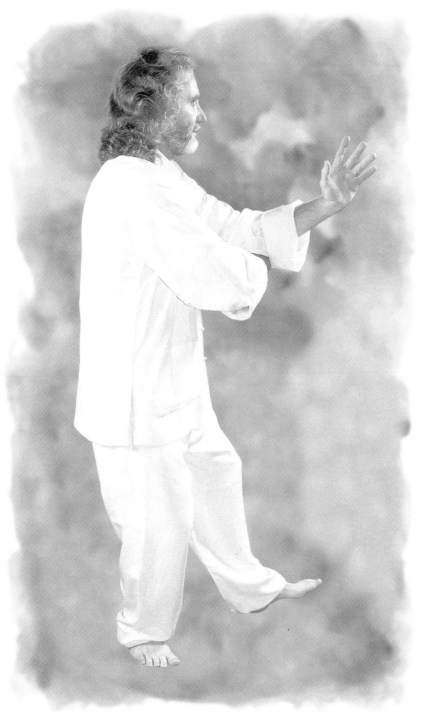

PICTURE 33

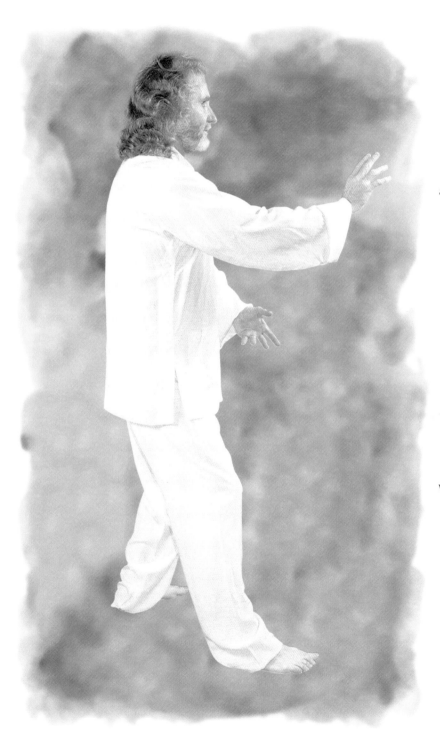

Step back and repulse monkey

Open both palms so that they both face up. Breathe in as you take your right palm back to the N.E. corner palm down, swing it firstly down in an arc and then up to shoulder height. Your body turns to the right slightly so that you are able to see the right palm. Take a step to the rear and to the S.E. with your left foot and place it so that the toe touches first. When the foot is placed it will have the toes pointing to the S.W. As your weight sits back the right palm comes past your ear as the left palm does an arc down to your left hip. The palms pass each other in the front of your body as you sit back. Exhale and turn your right toes to the West. The wrist remains relaxed until the final movement when it strikes and flexes. (Photo No. 34).

Step back and repulse monkey

(CONTINUES)

Next, turn your right palm over and now take your left palm back in the same way as you did with the right one, and Inhale. (Photo No. 35).

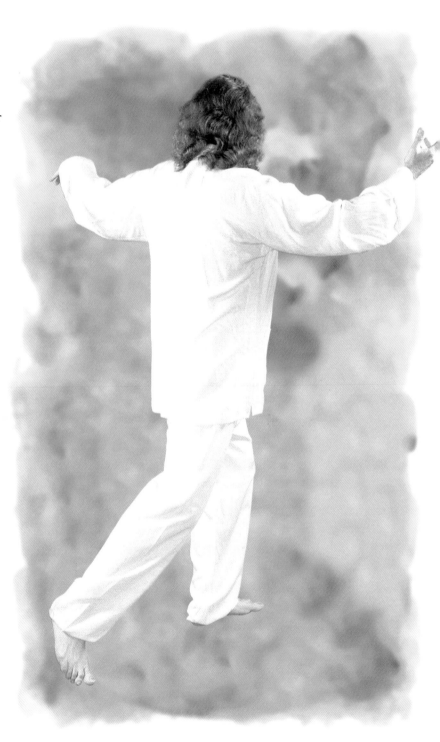

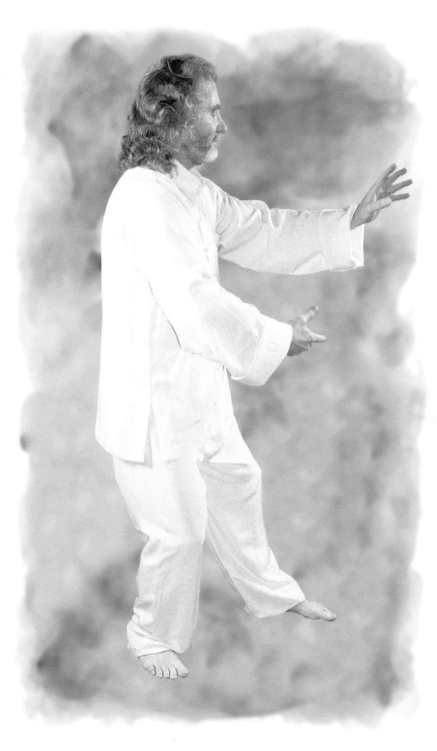

Step back and repulse monkey

(Continues)

Take a step with your right foot to the rear and as the weight goes back onto it the left palm strikes as the right palm blocks in the same way as before only reversed. Breathe out. (Photo No. 36). Turn the left palm over and repeat this on the right side again so that the right palm is striking as in Photo No. 34. Now repeat again on the left side so that the left palm is striking. (Photos 35 & 36). Now repeat again on the right and finish up with the right palm striking and the right foot forward still facing to the West. This is the same as Photo No. 34. You have now performed five `step back and repulse monkey' movements – right, left, right, left, right.

Stroking horse's mane

With the weight on your left leg, drop the right palm down and bring the left palm up on top to form the `ball posture', still facing to the West. Take a large step around to the N.E. corner with your right heel and place it into that corner. Now swivel on your heels as you change your weight onto the right foot, and cut up with your right arm as your left arm goes back down to your left side. Inhale when you hold the ball and exhale when you cut up. (Photo No. 37). Your right heel and your left toes should be on an East West line.

Lift hands

This is the same posture as in (Photo No. 16). This time you are facing a different direction to start. You lift both palms upward like wings, inhale and turn your left toes 45 degrees so that they point to the N.W. Place your weight onto the left leg, lift your palms to in front of you and exhale as you enter the `lift hands' posture.

PICTURE 37

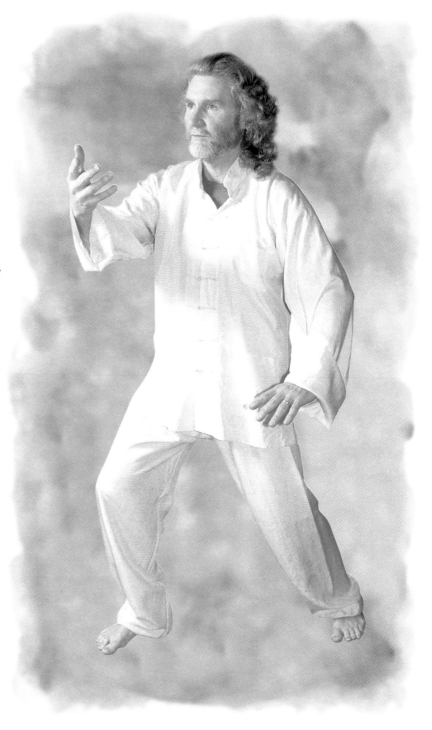

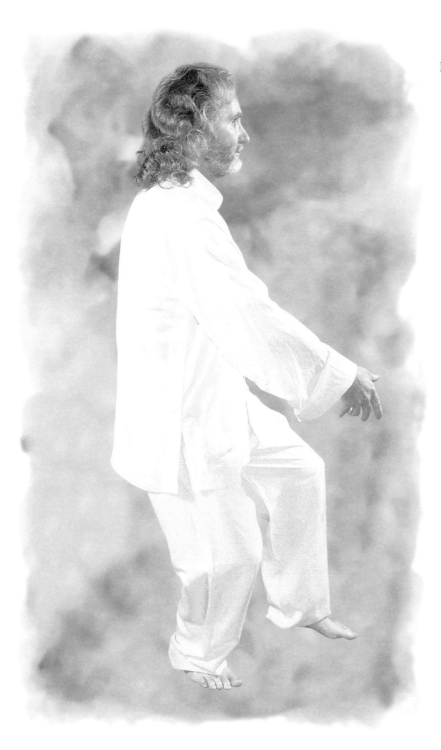

Pull down

This is the same as in Photo No. 17. The direction is also the same. Now repeat all movements from Photo No 18 to Photo No 21.

Golden needle at sea bottom

Pick up the right foot as in the first third and replace it in the same spot. As you inhale, the left foot is dragged slightly to the right to gain a `toe stance', as the body lowers so that the fingers of the right palm point to the ground. Exhale. Do not curve the back. (Photo No. 38). The eyes look straight ahead. Your left palm does not move.
Note: Keep your back vertical while performing this posture.

PICTURE 38

Fan through back

Inhale as you begin to lift your body up to the normal bent leg position and begin to take a left step forward. This also lifts your right palm up to a lateral position. The palm starts to turn over so that it is facing downwards. Take a step with your left foot diagonally and forward to the West (to the same position as for `brush knee twist step'). As your weight is placed onto your left foot the right palm pulls back facing away from your right ear while the left fingers poke upwards. Exhale.
(Photo No. 39).

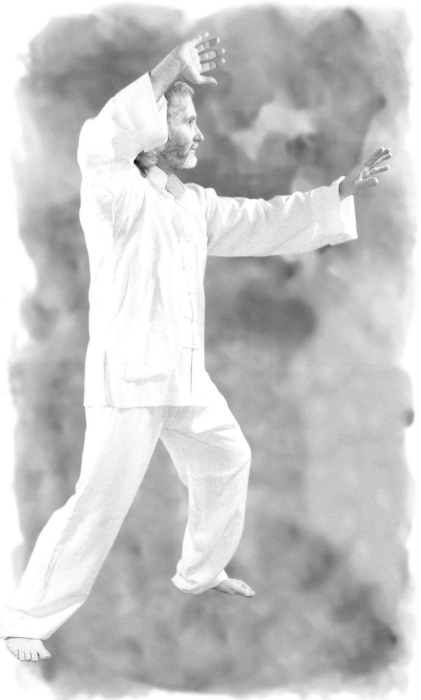

PICTURE 39

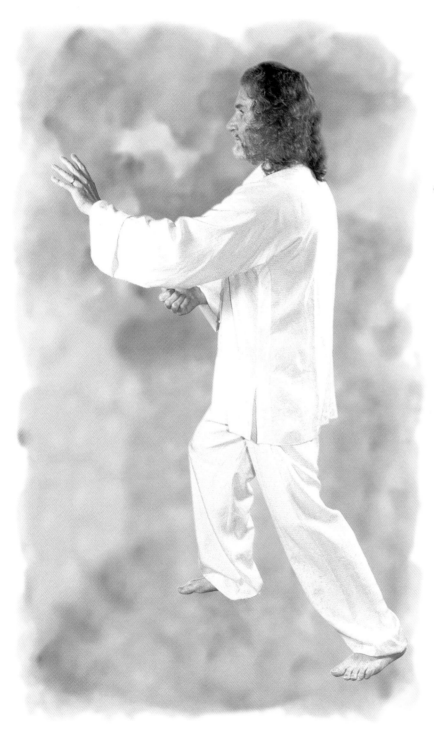

Turn around and chop with fist

A weighted turn, the left toes turn to the right by 90 degrees to face the North. At the same time make a fist with the right palm and bring it down in a clockwise circle until the thumb is pointing to the solar plexus. The left palm moves over your head to ward off, palm out. Inhale. Bring the right fist upwards to behind the left palm, at the same time step with your right foot to the East. Chop downwards with the right fist until it arrives at your right hip and the left palm attacks to the East. The weight is on the right leg. Exhale. (Photo No. 40).

PICTURE 40

Upper cut, step forward, parry and punch

The right fist punches straight up to end directly in front of the left palm which has not moved. (No breath). The fist now turns down (palm facing down) as the left palm turns up. Inhale as both palms come down to your left side and up to your left ear, as your right foot picks up and is placed down again in front, turning only 45 degrees to the S.E. The left palm is attacking while the right is at your right hip. Exhale. Now you should step to the East this time and inhale. As the weight comes down onto your left leg you perform a straight punch as in Photo No. 26. Exhale.

Diagonal P'eng

Your left palm slides under your right forearm. Both palms are facing down. Keeping the weight on your left leg you turn your left toes to the N.E. and slide your left palm out to that corner. (Photo No. 41).

PICTURE 41

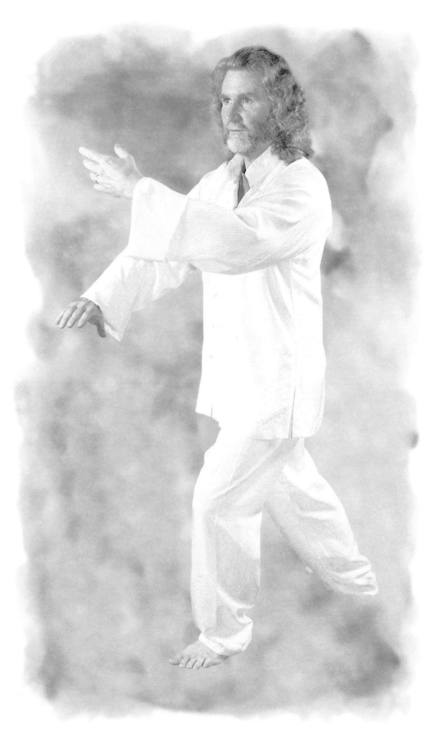

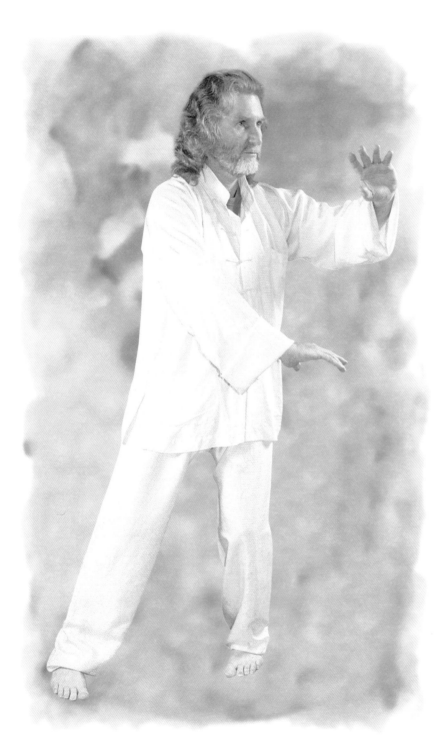

Grasping swallow's tail

Now we perform these same postures again. Firstly, bring the right palm under your left palm and inhale as in Photo No. 7, only you begin in a slightly different step. Now step to the East with your right foot for Double p'eng as in Photo No. 8. Pull back, as in Photo No. 9. Chee as in Photo No. 10. Sit back as in Photo No. 11. Press as in Photo No. 12. Sit back ready as in Photo No. 13. Fishes in eight as in Photo 14. Single whip as in Photo No.15.

N.B. Whenever we cexecute this sequence, I will say,repeat `grasping swallow's tail' up to `single whip'.

Wave hands like clouds

Turn the left foot to point to the North, a weighted turn. Inhale. At the same time, bring the right palm across in front of your forehead and into the N.W. corner, and flex your right palm and bring it down and across in an arc to directly under the left palm. (Photo No. 42).

PICTURE 42

Wave hands like clouds

(CONTINUED)

Push the left palm down on the outside of the right one with the palm facing downward while the right one comes up the inside as if rubbing your stomach. Simultaneously, the right foot is dragged back to parallel as you exhale. (Photo No. 43). Body still facing to the N.W.

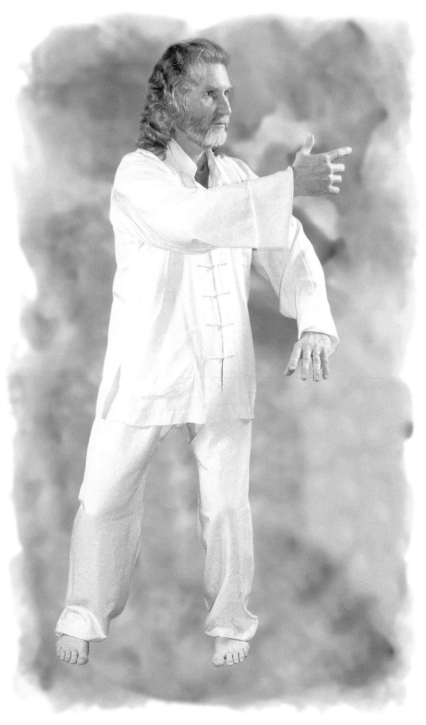

PICTURE 43

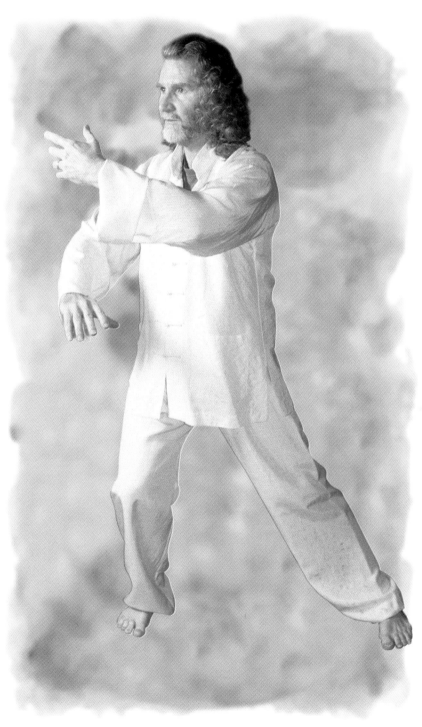

Wave hands like clouds

(Continued)

NB: I am giving this to you in the static way but this movement, as with all of them is done flowingly. Turn your torso to the N.E. and change your weight to your right leg. Change hands as before, only reversed i.e. the right palm pushes down as the left palm rubs the stomach, as you breathe in and take a double shoulder width step to your left. (Photo No. 44).
NB: This is your second step, counting the first time that you pulled the right foot back. There are nine steps and palm changes to make.

PICTURE 44

Wave hands like clouds

(CONTINUED)

Turn your torso to the N.W. corner holding your palms in that same position, left up and right down. Now, change your palms again, left down and right up as you drag your right foot up to single shoulder width as you exhale. (Photo No. 45).

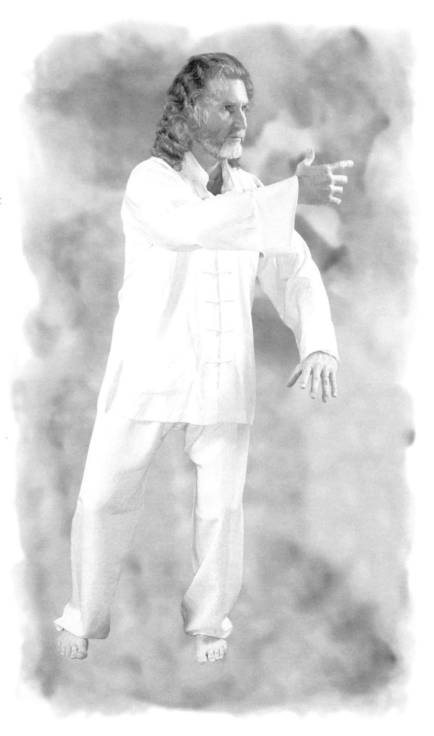

PICTURE 45

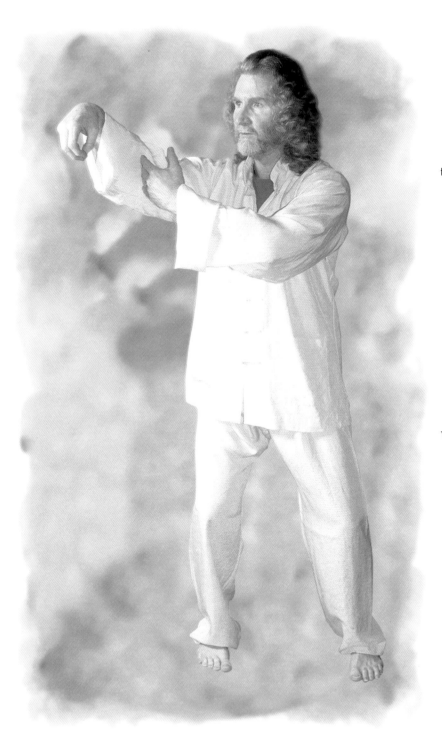

Wave hands like clouds

(CONTINUED)

This is your third step. Your right palm is now on the top. From here you repeat the turn to the N.E. and the change with the step, (4th step). (Photo No. 44). Turn to the N.W., step and change, (5th step). (Photo No. 45). Turn to the N.E., step and change, (6th step). (Photo No. 44. Turn to the N.W., step and change, (7th step). (Photo No. 45). Turn to the N.E., step and change, (8th step). (Photo No. 44). Turn to the N.W., step and change, (9th step). (Photo No. 45). This was your last step, you now turn back to the N.E., with your right palm on the top and bring your left palm up with the fingers pointing in to the inside of your right elbow. (Photo No. 46). Inhale.

PICTURE **46**

Single whip

From this position you now perform `single whip' exactly as before, (Photo No.15). You are now facing to the West.

Lifting up the heavens

From `single whip', sit back onto your right leg and turn both palms upward as if holding two plates. Inhale. (Photo No. 47).

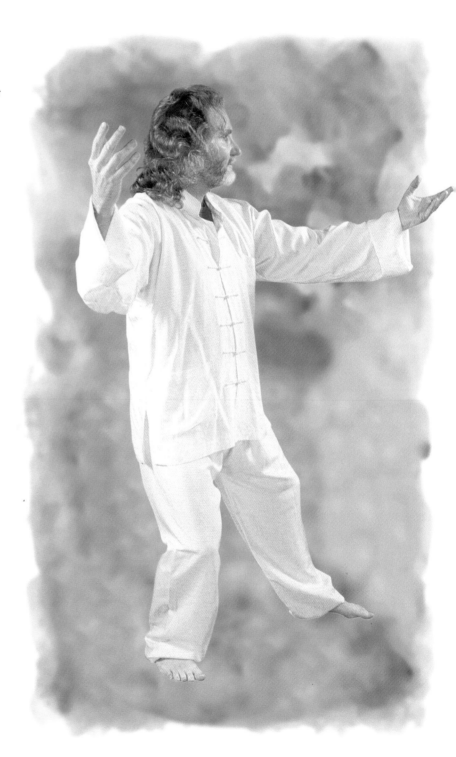

PICTURE 47

High pat on horse

The right palm pushes past your right ear, with the fingers pointing in to the ear, and attacks to the West. At the same time the left palm does a clockwise arc down the front of your body to end up at your left hip. The left foot is dragged back and makes a toe stance as you exhale. (Photo No. 48).

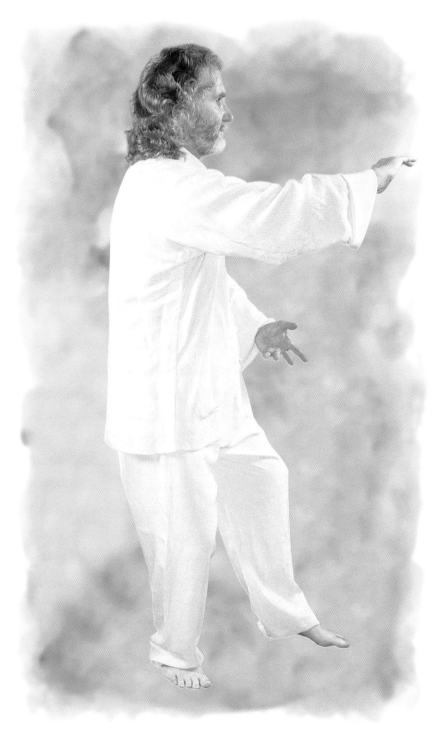

Drawing the bow
(RIGHT)

Cross your right palm over your left forearm. The right palm is facing down while the left is up. The circle continues with both hands making clockwise circles 180 degrees out of sync. The left palm crosses over the inside of your right forearm. As this is happening the left foot takes a step to the S.W. corner as you inhale. Now, as the weight is transferred to your left foot, the left palm is pulled back to your left ear as the right palm attacks into the N.W. corner as if drawing a bow. Exhale. (Photo No. 49).

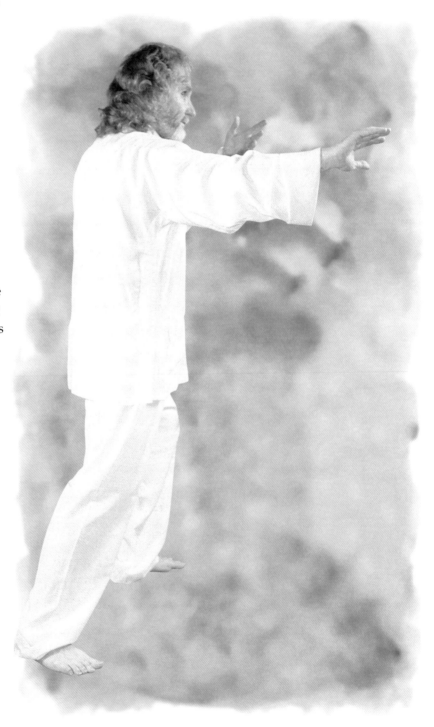

PICTURE 49

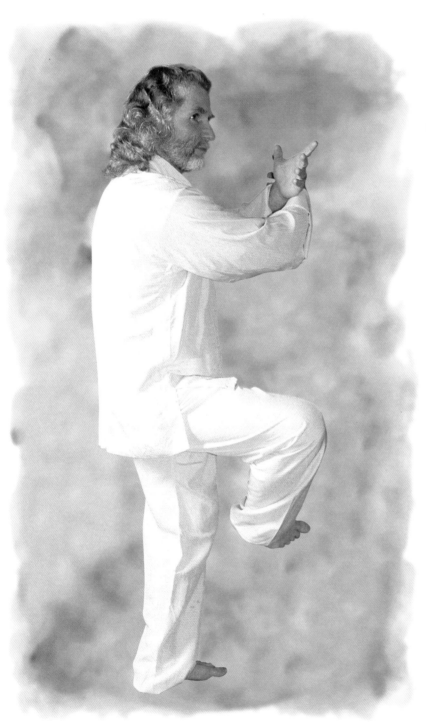

Separation of right leg

(RIGHT INSTEP KICK)

Move your right palm down in an arc across your body and up to cross over your left forearm, palms towards you. As your arms come up to cross, your right foot comes up as you inhale. (Photo No. 50).

PICTURE 50

Separation of right leg

(CONTINUED)

Turn your palms outward as you push both palms out to the South (left) and N.W. (right). Straighten your left leg as this happens and exhale. As soon as your arms are in position and your left leg is straight, you kick your left foot out to the N.W. corner as you inhale. Note that the foot and hand should not reach out together, nor should there be a long wait before the foot kicks. The foot reaches its goal a split second after the right palm is in position. (Photo No.51).

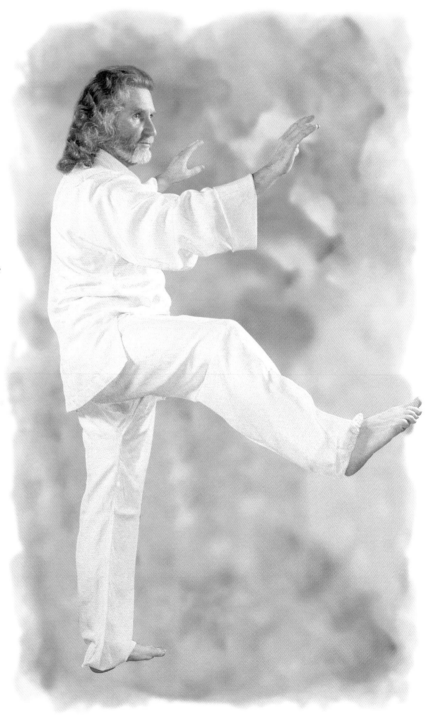

PICTURE 51

68

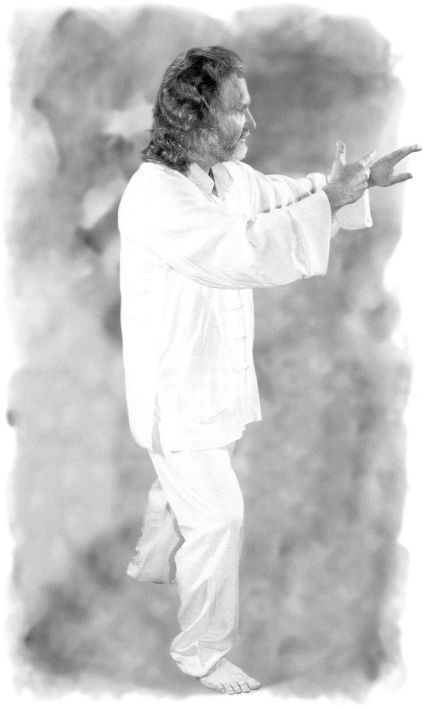

Drawing the bow
(LEFT)

From the last position, turn
your right palm over and as
you step to the N.W. corner
your left palm circles in to
touch the inside of your right
elbow. This happens as the
right heel touches the ground.
Now the left palm circles out to
form the drawing bow posture
exactly as before only reversed.
Exhale on the down step and
up to the bow. (Photo No. 52).

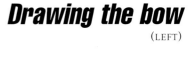

PICTURE **52**

Separation of left leg

(LEFT INSTEP KICK)

As before, only opposite, cross the arms in front of you and open the palms out to the S.W. (left) and to the N. (right) and perform the kick with the instep of the left foot. Inhale. (Inhale is correct as this is an upward movement!) (Photo No. 53). On the completion of this kick the left foot is brought back in to the right knee which has bent downward again, the arms are as they were for the kick. Exhale.

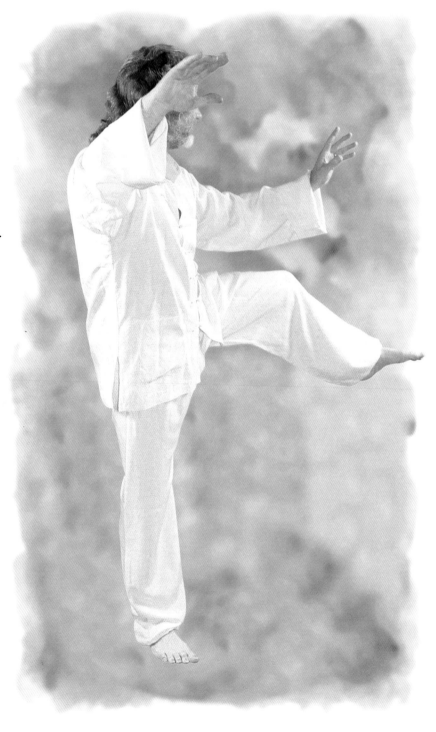

PICTURE 53

Spin around and kick with heel

You must now use your left foot as the lever to spin you around on your right heel so that your right toes point to the South and your arms are crossed at the last with the natural flow of the movement. The left toes are off the ground and your body is facing to the S.E. (Photo No. 54).

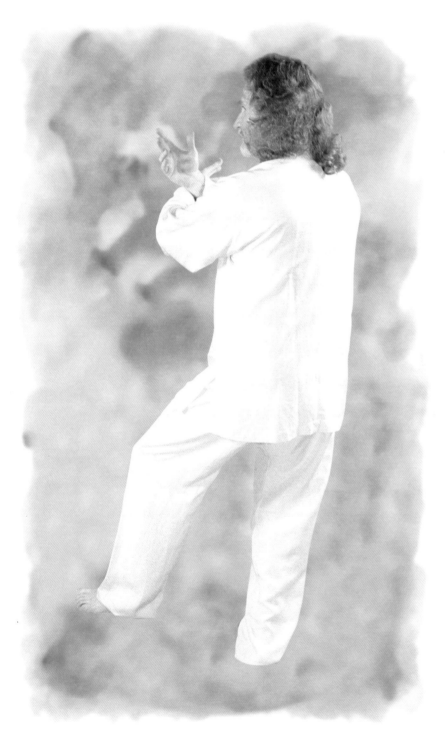

PICTURE **54**

Spin around and kick with heel

(CONTINUED)

Still on that last out breath you now lift your left knee as your palms open out and push out as before. (All of the kicks start the same). Breathe in as you kick with your left heel to the E. (Photo No.55).

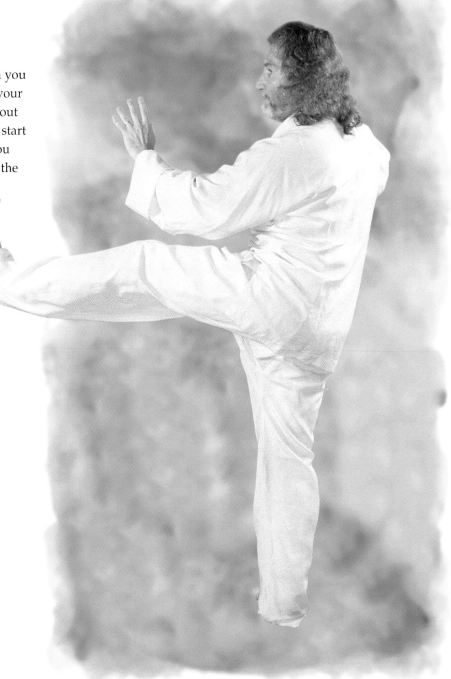

PICTURE **55**

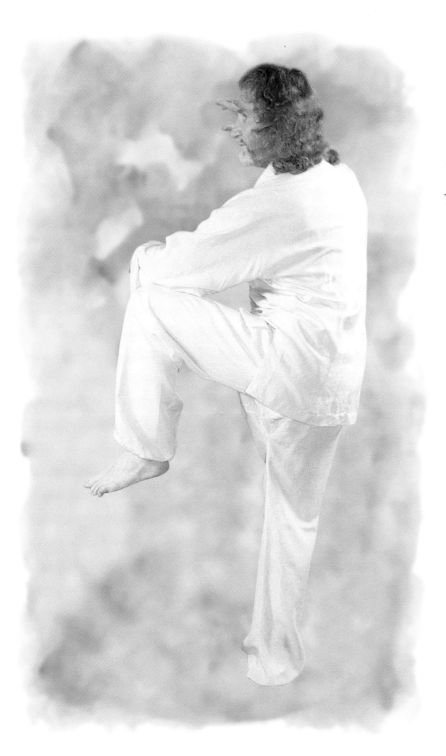

Spin around and kick with heel

(CONTINUED)

Finish by bending your right leg and laying your left elbow across your left knee, the right palm relaxes. (Photo No. 56). This is part of your out-breath.

PICTURE 56

Brush knee twist step

Brush your left knee with your left palm as you step to the E. with your left foot and push with your right palm as you exhale. Your right toes come around by 45 degrees. (Photo No. 57).

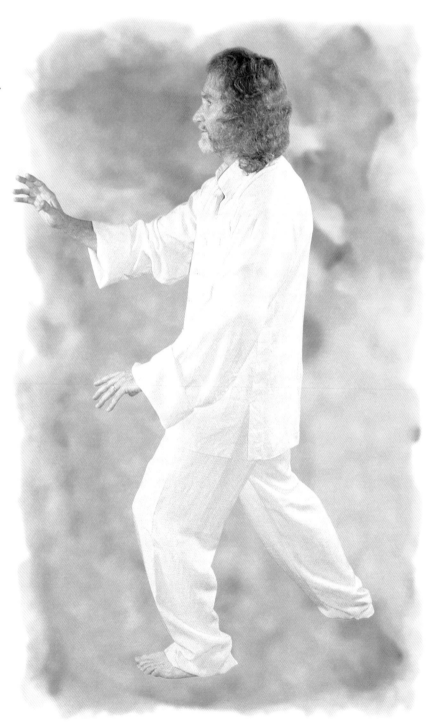

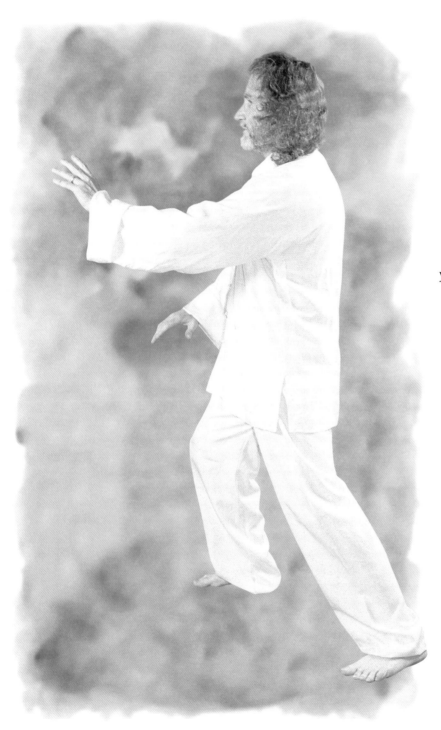

Brush knee twist step
(RIGHT)

Now you must perform brush knee twist step exactly as you performed it in the first third. Turn the left foot out by 45 degrees to the N.E. and hold the ball on the left with the right palm on the top. Brush your right knee and step with the right knee to the East as you attack with your left palm. (Photo No. 58).

PICTURE 58

Strike The Tri-Points

Some teachers call this posture "punch to knee". Turn your right foot 45 degrees to the S.E. and place your fist onto your right knee. You must bend slightly for this but do not curve your back. The left palm comes over as if holding the ball. Inhale. (Photo No. 59).

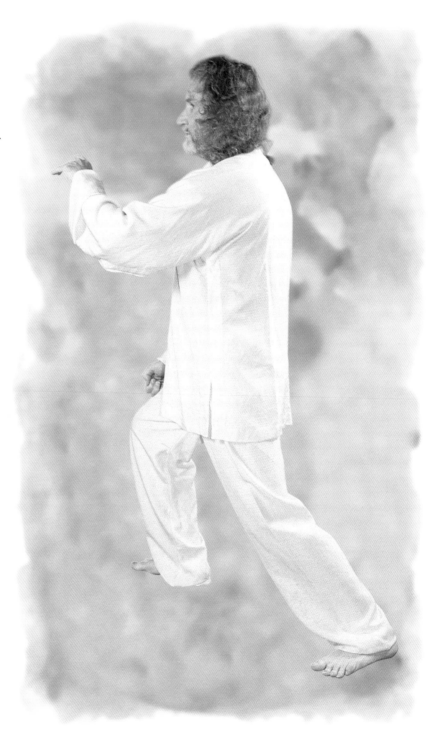

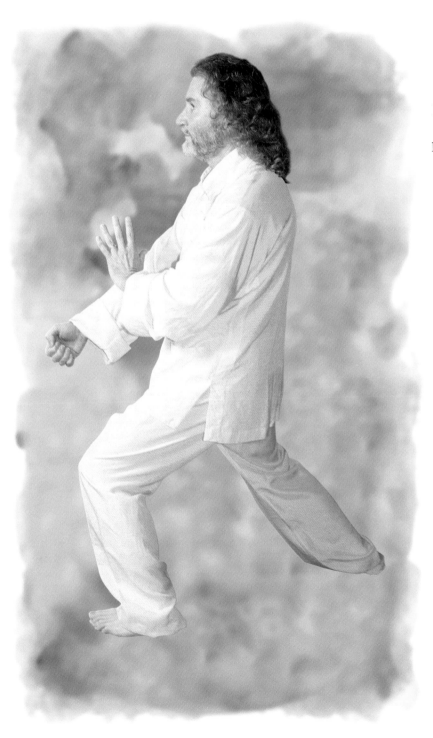

Strike The Tri-Points
(CONTINUED)

Facing the East, step to the East with your left foot and as the knee comes through, brush it as if for brush knee twist step. As the weight comes down onto the left foot, the right fist naturally comes forward and swings forward. Exhale. (Photo No. 60).

Turn around and chop with fist

Exactly the same movement with the same name as before, only starting from a different position. Inhale as your right fist comes up to your solar plexus and your left foot does a weighted turn so that the toes point to the South. Your left palm comes up to strike overhead. You will end up this time facing to the West, attacking with your left palm and right foot forward. (Photo No. 40). Exhale.

PICTURE 60

Uppercut, step forward, parry and punch

Exactly the same as before only the direction is to the West. Punch up and turn the left palm over with the right fist down. This is still part of the last exhalation. Pull down to your left, bring both palms up to your ear and inhale. Punch down with the back of your right fist across your body as you strike with your left palm to the West. (Photo No. 25). Step through to the West with your left foot and punch with your right fist. Exhale. (Photo No. 26).

Diagonal P'eng

The same as before only to the S.W. Slide your left palm under your right wrist and p'eng into the S.W. corner as your left foot swivels to the S.W. The right palm comes down to your right side. The only difference this time is that you now look at your right palm as it strikes. (Photo No. 61).

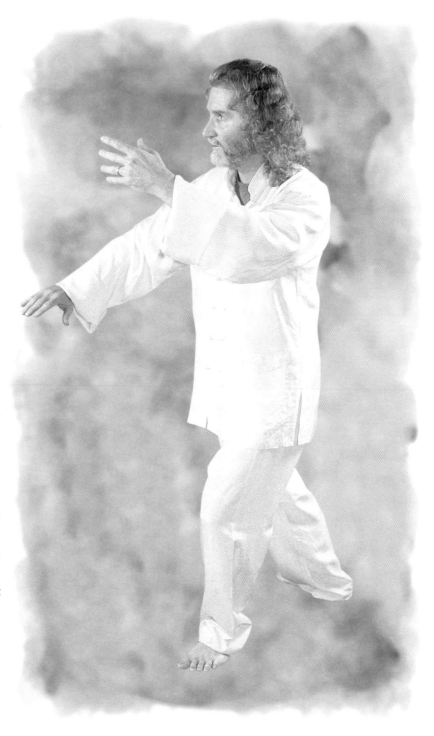

PICTURE 61

Right heel kick

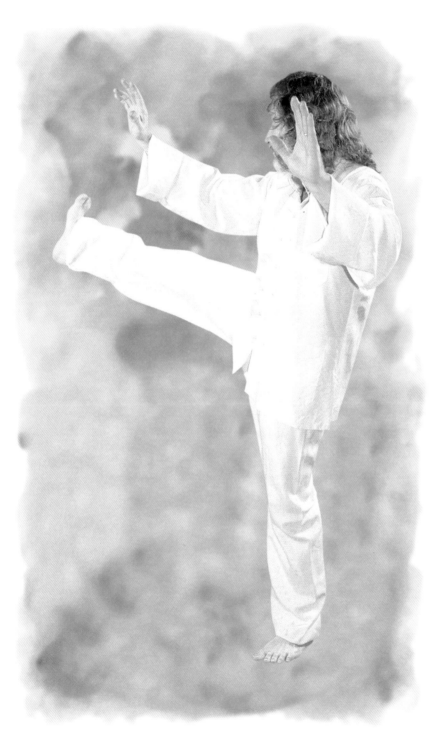

Circle your right arm back up to be across the left forearm as for any of the kicks. Inhale. Push both palms out to the North West (right) and South (left) as you kick to the N.W. with your right heel. Exhale as you push your palms out and in as you kick. (Photo No. 62).

PICTURE 62

Attack
to the right

Exhale as you put the right foot down exactly parallel to the left foot and point the right thumb to your breastbone. Leave the left palm as for the kick. You are now facing to the S.W. corner and your feet are on the S.E. to N.W. diagonal. (Photo No. 63).

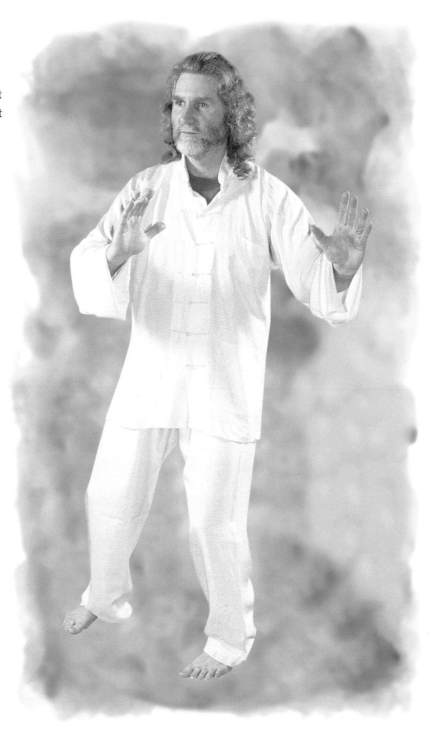

PICTURE 63

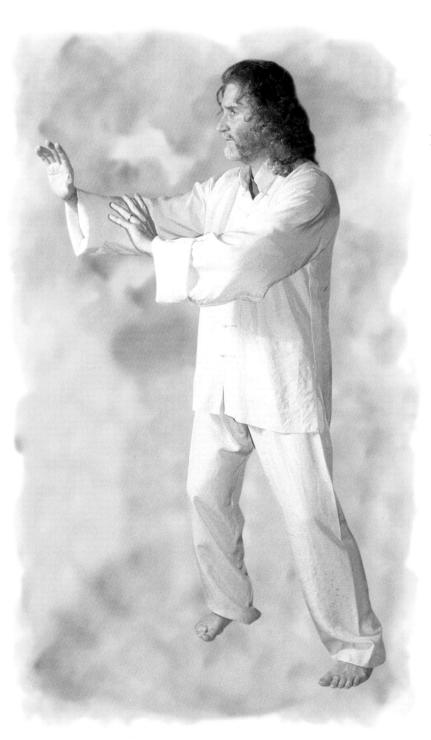

Attack
to the right
(CONTINUED)

Continue the out breath as you push the right palm to the West and change the weight to the right foot. The left palm comes across to where the right one was. (Photo No. 64).

Hit tiger left

Turn the left palm over and step to the S.E. corner with the left foot as you inhale. As the weight rolls on to the left foot, bring the left palm across your body to the left and form fists with both palms. Exhale as you punch. The right toes are dragged around by 45 degrees to point to the South.
(Photo No. 65).

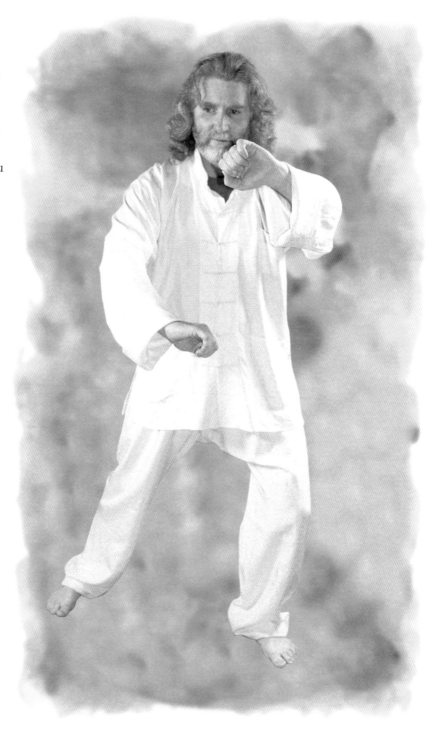

PICTURE 65

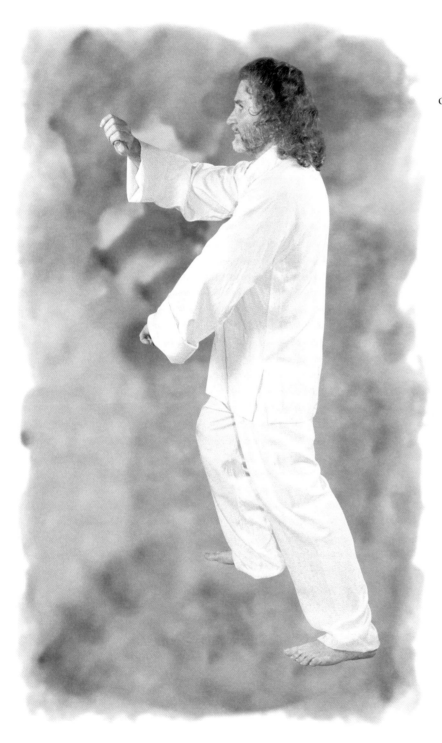

Hit tiger right

Turn the left toes 90 degrees to the S.W., a weighted turn, and open the right palm to palm up. The left palm simultaneously wards off at the left temple. It simply opens so that the palm is facing outward. Inhale. Lift the right foot and put it down into the N.W. corner. As you roll onto it, bring your right palm down and across your body as before. When your right palm is parallel to the ground, form two fists and strike as before only the right fist is on top. Exhale. (Photo No. 66).

PICTURE **66**

Phoenix punch and turn

Still on that last out breath, bring the left fist up to join the right fist as you simultaneously turn your left foot to the South and change your weight onto it as you drag your right toes around to point to the S.W. (Photo No. 67).

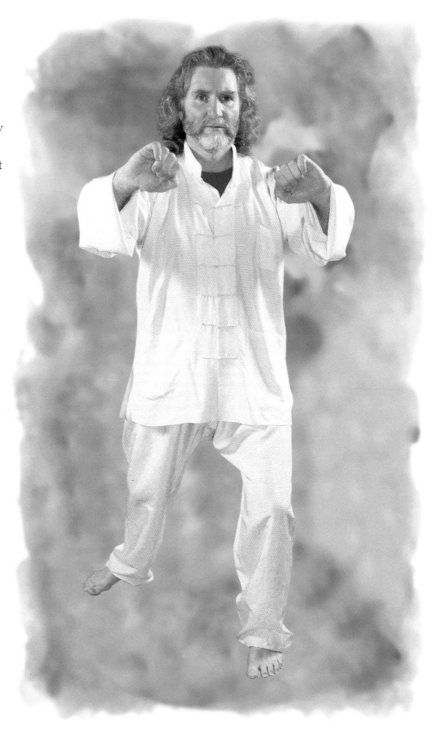

PICTURE 67

Kick with right heel

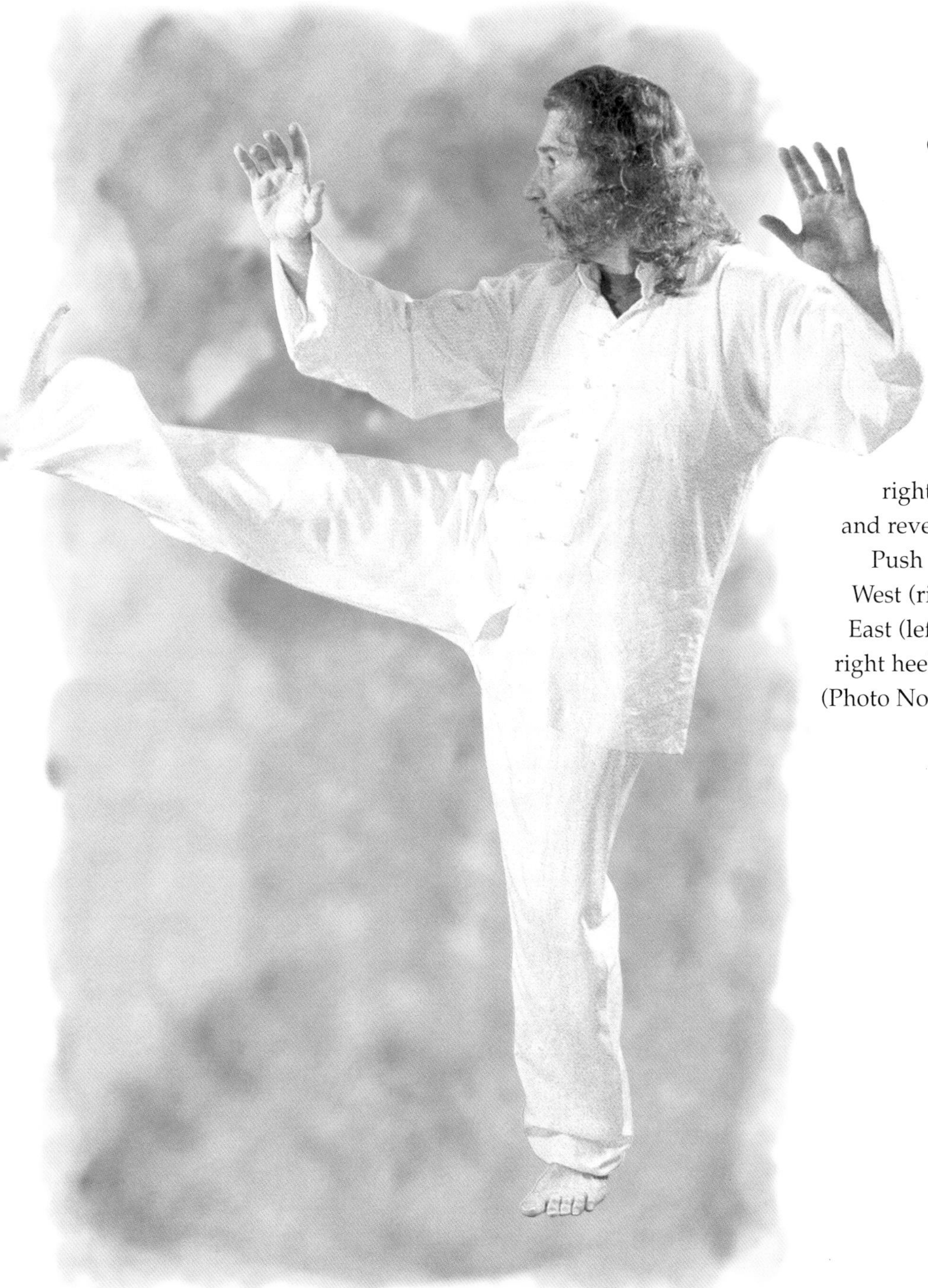

Open both palms and circle them out and down as you inhale. Bring both palms back up to cross in front as for all of the kicks, right palm on the outside. (If you kick with the right foot, right palm on the outside, and reversed for the left foot). Push both palms out to the West (right) and to the South East (left) and kick with your right heel to the West. Same as (Photo No. 68) only to the West.

PICTURE 68

Double wind goes through ears

From that last kick, turn both palms over and brush the outside of your right knee. (Photo No. 69).

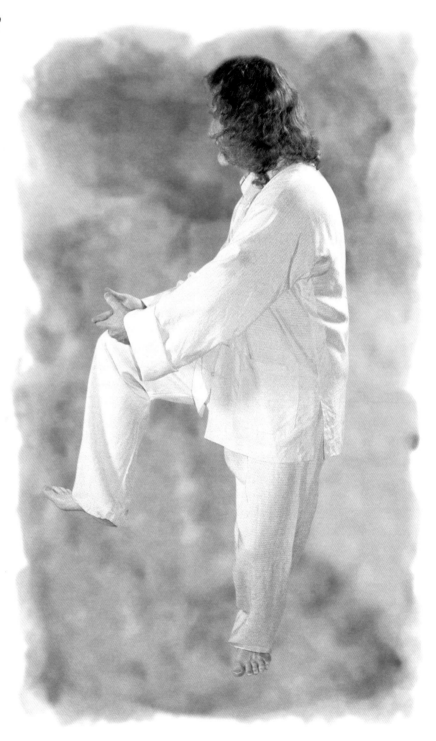

PICTURE 69

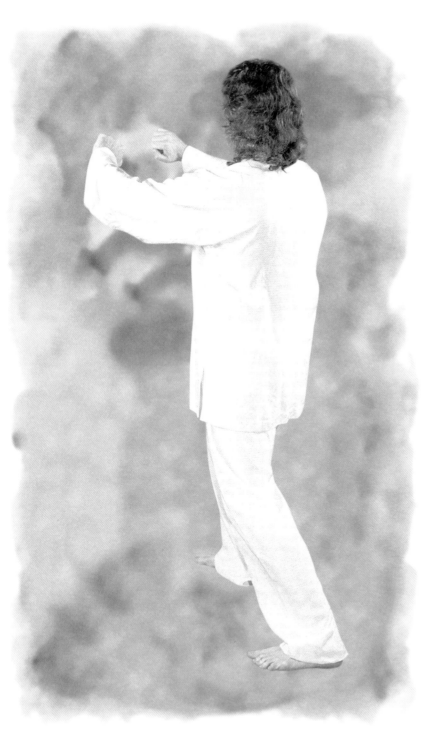

Double wind goes through ears

(Continued)

As you step down into the N.W. corner and perform this posture. Exhale. Both palms sweep downward and circle back up making fists as this happens. (Photo No. 70). The left foot is dragged around by 90 degrees to point into the West. The right foot points to the N.W.

Left heel kick

Open both palms and circle them to cross left over right ready for the kick. As before, push both palms out and kick with your left heel to the West.

Spin around and kick

Use your left leg as a lever and throw it to your right to cause you to spin around on the ball of your right foot. Your left foot lands with the weight being placed upon it to the rear with the toes pointing to the S.W. You are still facing to the W. as your palms cross in front of you, right over left.
(Photo No. 71).

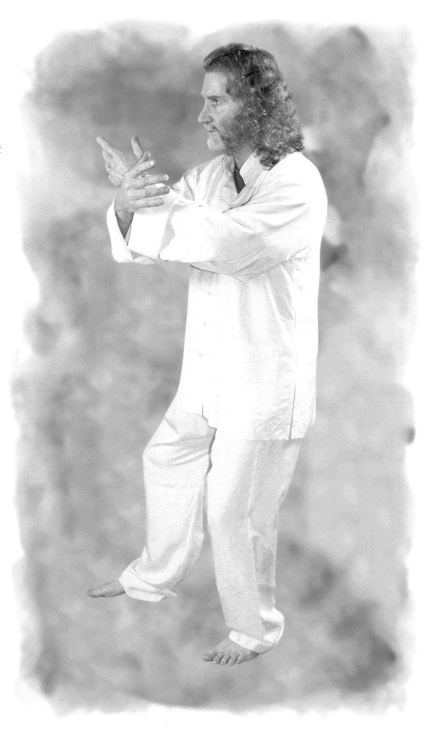

PICTURE 71

Right heel kick

Open both palms as before and kick to the N.W. with your right heel as you inhale. (Photo No. 72).

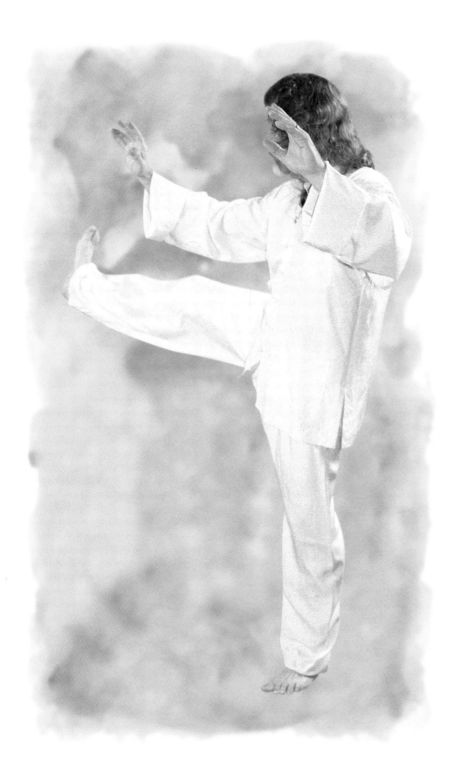

Step up parry and punch

Exactly as before when you finished the first third. From the last kick, place your right elbow onto your right knee. (Photo No. 73). Exhale as you circle your right fist up to your left ear and repeat as for Photo No. 25. (Left palm strike weighted on your right foot turned to the N.W.) Step through and punch with your right fist. (Photo No. 26).

Sit back and press forward.

As in photos Nos. 27 and 28.

Apparent close up.

As in photo No. 47.

This is the end of the second third. The beginning of the final third is exactly the same as before.

PICTURE 73

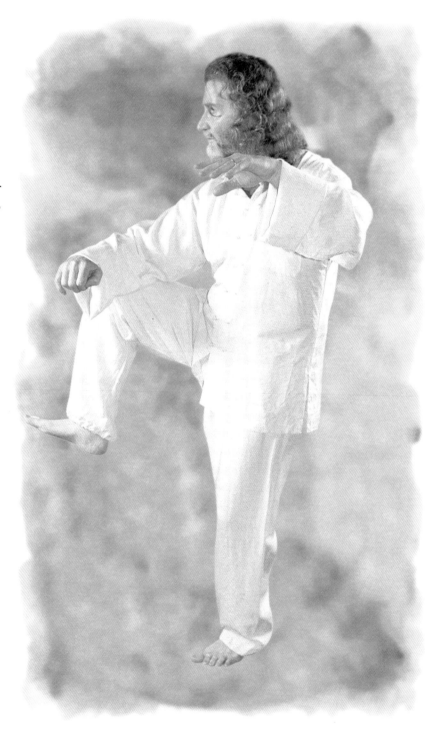

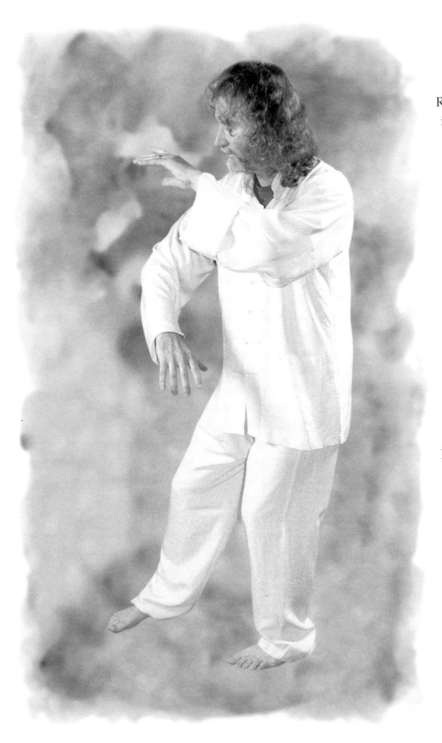

Starting the final third

Repeat: **Embrace tiger return to mountain** and **Raise your right palm.** (Photo Nos. 30 and 31), then repeat from **Pull back** through to **Sit back ready** (Photo Nos. 9-13). These postures should be to the Southeast and not to the East. Then perform **Fishes in eight** (Photo No. 14) to the North, and then to the East, and **Single whip** (to the North West) the same way as before. (Photo No.15).

Slant Flying
(RIGHT)

From `single whip' to the N.W., turn your left toes (a weighted turn) 90 degrees to point to the N.E. At the same time hold a ball with your right palm under. (Photo No. 74).

PICTURE 74

Slant flying

(RIGHT CONTINUED)

Inhale. Take a step into the S.E.
corner with your right foot, the
toes of which point to the S.W.
As you change your weight
onto the right foot, exhale as
you cut up with your right
palm and down with your left
palm. Your right wrist is in
your centre while your right
elbow is over your right knee.
Your left toes turn to the East.
(Photo No. 75).

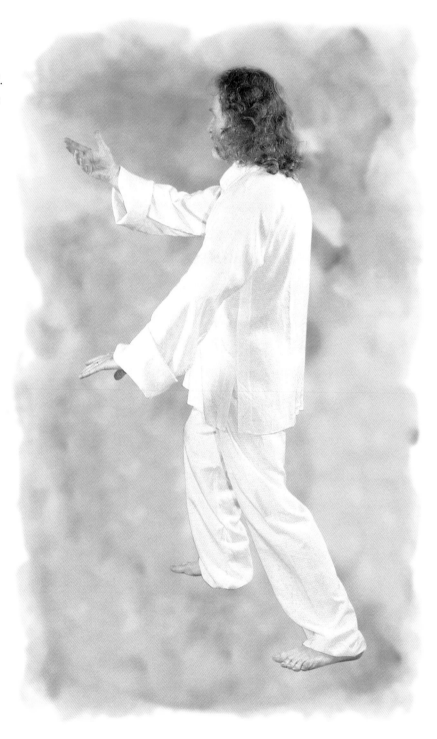

PICTURE 75

Slant flying

From the last position, turn
your right toes to the South
(weighted) as you breathe in
and hold the ball with your
right palm on the top.
(Photo No. 76).

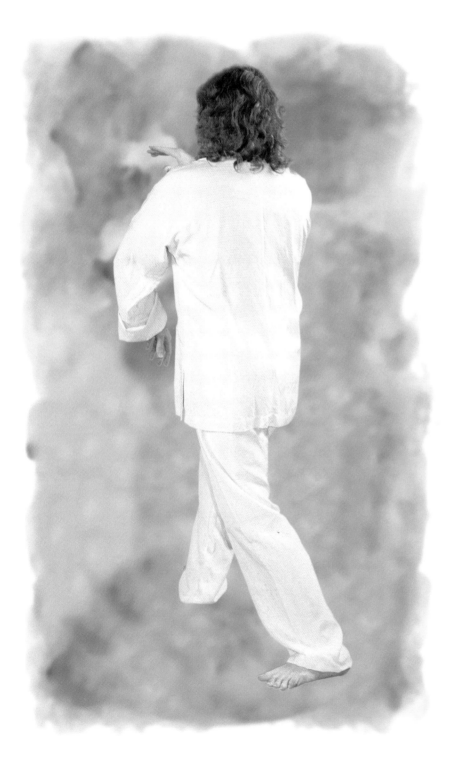

PICTURE 76

Slant flying

(Left Continued)

Now as before, only to the opposite direction, step to the N.E. corner with your left foot and as the weight is transferred onto your right foot, slant upward with your left palm as your right one goes back down to your right side and your right toes are dragged around to the East. Exhale.
(Photo No. 77).

Slant flying

(Right)

As before, hold the ball with your left palm on the top and turn your left toes to the North as you inhale. Step to the S.E. corner with your right foot and perform `slant flying' again into that corner as before.
(Photo No. 75).

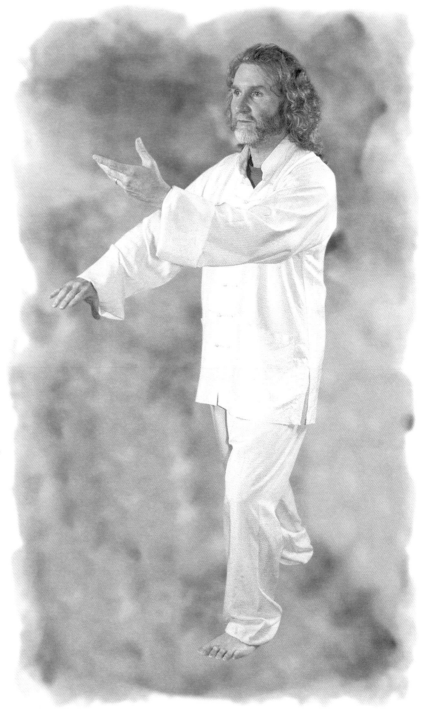

PICTURE 77

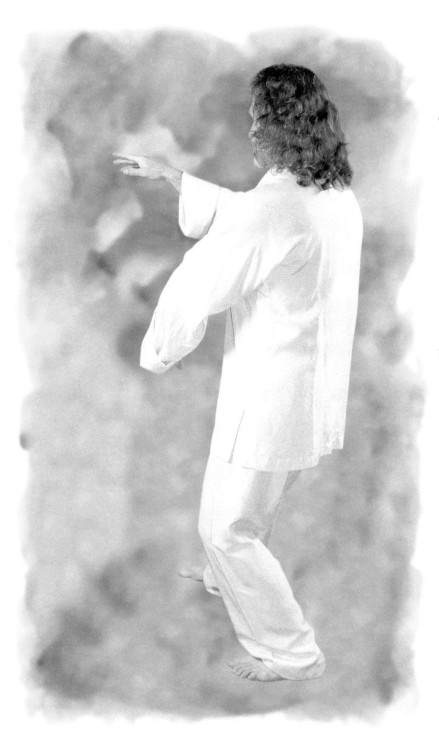

Sit back and block

From the last position, sit back onto your left foot and block as in Photo No. 78. Inhale. Turn your right toes 90 degrees to the N.E. and then put your weight onto that leg. You are now facing to the N.E.

Grasping swallow's tail

This is exactly as in the beginning. (Photos 6, 7, 8, 9, 10, 11, 12). Repeat again all of the postures up to and including single whip. (Photos 13, 14,15).

PICTURE 78

Fair lady works at shuttles

From single whip to the West (the directions for the last set of movements were also exactly the same as in the beginning), do a weighted turn on your left heel so that your toes point to the North. As you do this, hold a ball, with your left palm under. Inhale. (Photo No. 79).

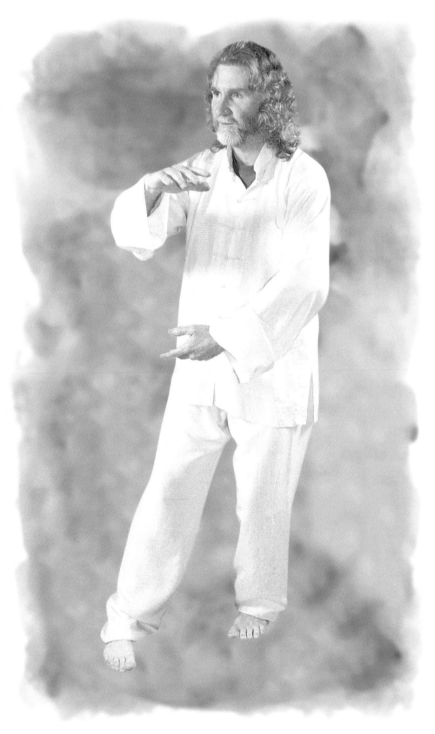

PICTURE 79

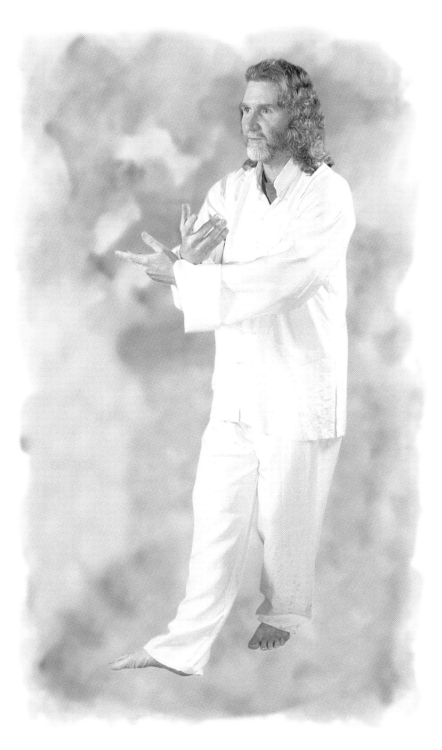

Fair lady works at shuttles

(Continued)

As your wrists cross (palms upward), your right foot is picked up and is placed down again with the toes pointing to the East. (Photo No.80).

Fair lady works at shuttles

(CONTINUED)

Take a step to the N.E. corner with your left foot (toes to the N.E.) and as your left heel touches, your right palm is dragged down to your right hip as your left palm wards off over head. (Photo No. 81).

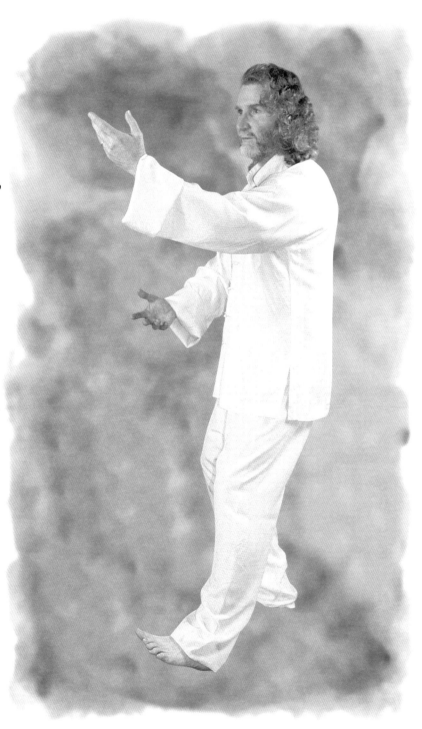

PICTURE **81**

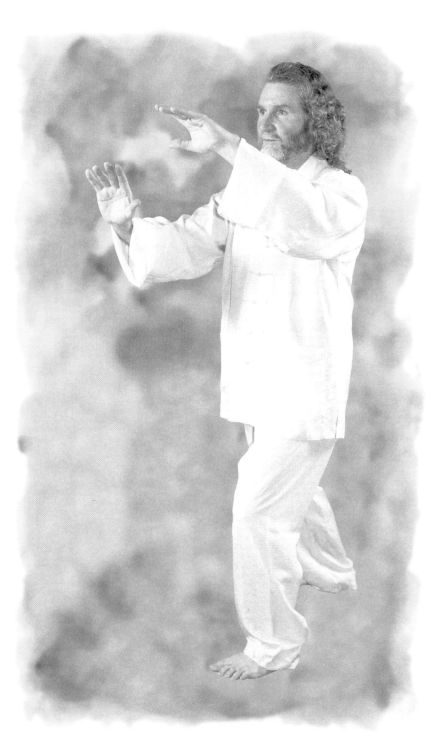

Fair lady works at shuttles
(CONTINUED)

Now, change your weight to your left leg as your right palm comes up and strikes into the N.E. corner. Exhale. (Photo No. 82).

PICTURE 82

Fair lady works at shuttles

(Continued)

From here you have to repeat this posture into the N.W. corner. Firstly, push downward with your right palm as your left toes turn right around to point to the South (weighted). Breathe in as you hold a ball with the right palm under. (Photo No. 83).

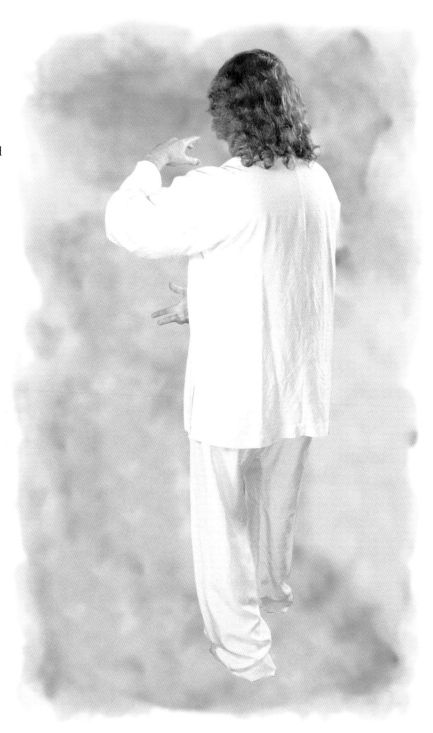

PICTURE 83

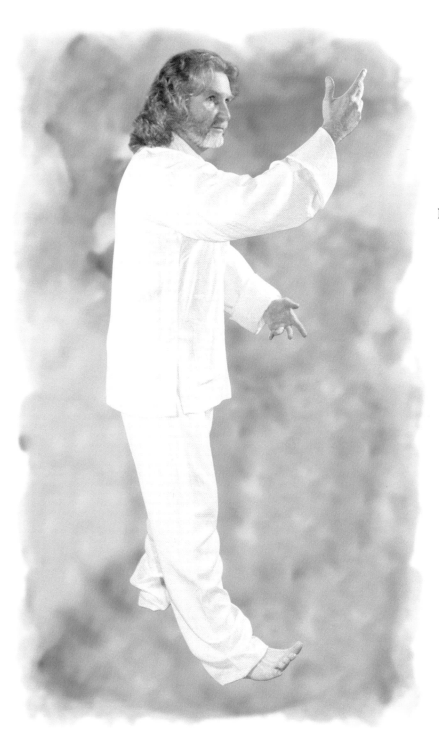

Fair lady works at shuttles

(CONTINUED)

Cross your wrists as before only with the right under and step into the N.W. corner, as your left palm comes down to your left side and your right palm wards off. (Photo No. 84).

PICTURE 84

Fair lady works at shuttles

(CONTINUED)

Roll your weight onto your right foot as your left palm strikes, with weight still on your right leg. (Photo No. 85).

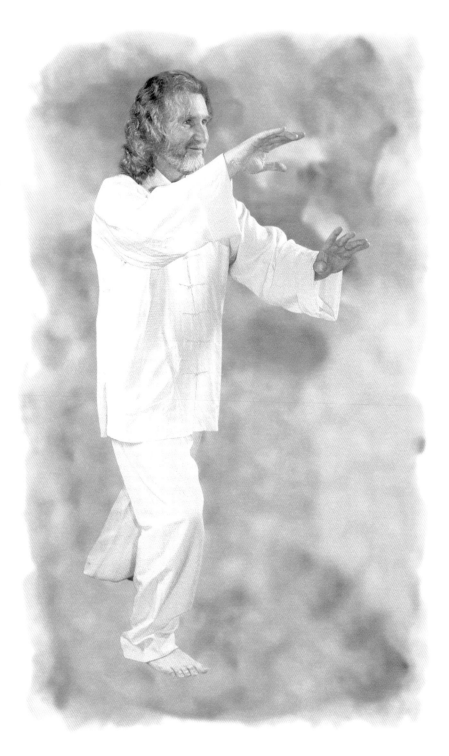

PICTURE 85

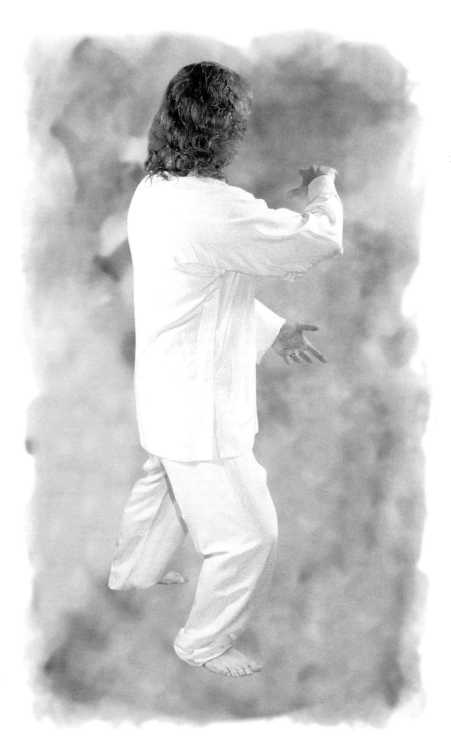

Hold a ball, left palm under

Cross your wrists as before, left under and step into the S.W. corner with your left foot, as your right palm comes down to your right side and your left palm wards off. (Photo No. 86).

Hold a ball, left palm under

(CONTINUED)

Roll onto your left leg as you strike with your right palm. (Photo No. 87). (S.W.)

Now you must repeat exactly the same movements as in photos 82, 83 and 84. You have now performed 'fair lady works at shuttles' into the four corners starting with the N.E. then the N.W. then the S.W. and the S.E.

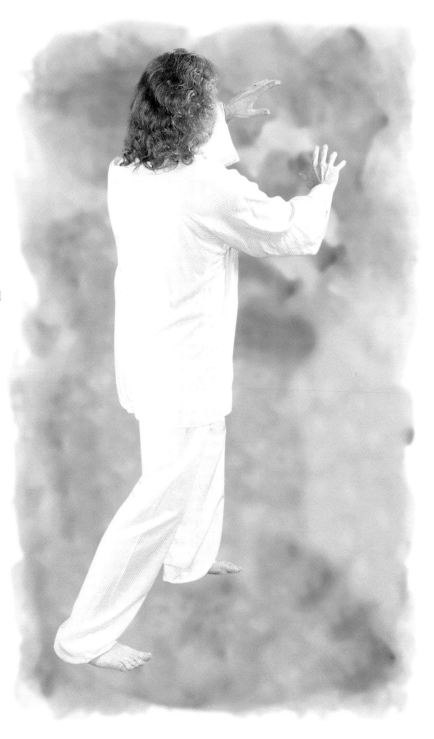

PICTURE 87

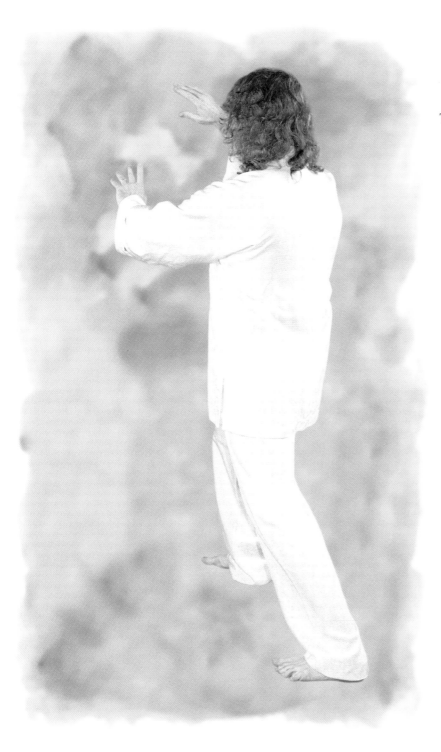

Hold a ball, left palm under

(CONTINUED)

The last set of movements went from the S.W. corner into the S.E. corner but the photos are the same as from the N.E. corner to the N.W. corner. You finish up as in Photo No. 88. Repeat photo No. 78, then repeat photos 6, 7, 8, 9, 10, 11, 12. Now repeat Photo Nos. 13 and 14. Finally repeat Photo No.25.

PICTURE 88

Wave hands in clouds

Exactly the same way that you performed these postures in the second third. Repeat photos 42, 43, 44, 45, 46.

Single whip

Repeat Photo No.15.

Snake creeps down

Turn your right toes to the N.E. then the heel is turned out with toes pointing N.W. The toes are again turned to the N.E. to achieve a wider stance. Inhale. Drop down onto your right leg so that the knee of the right leg is over the right toes, the left foot has adjusted itself so that the toes point to the N.W. with both feet flat on the ground. You breathe in as you shuffle backwards and out as you drop down. The right palm stays as for single whip, while the left drops. (Photo No. 89).

PICTURE 89

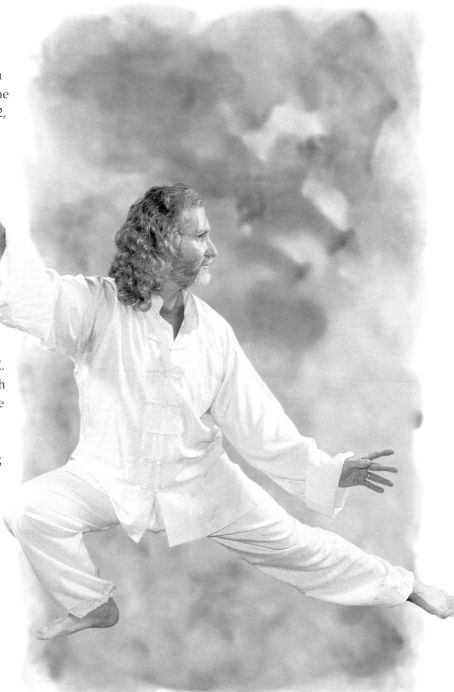

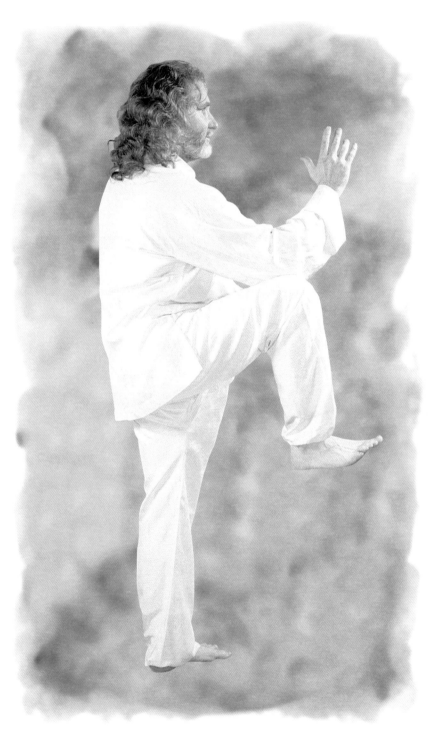

Golden cock stands on one leg
(LEFT)

As you bring your weight onto your left leg, turn your left toes out by 90 degrees to point to the S.W. The toes of the right foot are dragged forwards so that they point to the N.W. The left palm is as if poking forwards while the fingers of the right palm open up. Continuing, bring your right palm downward in an arc and as it comes up, stand up in one sweep. Don't drag the toes on the ground, the right foot should turn as much as possible to allow for this. Bring your right elbow up onto your right knee and your left palm goes back down to your left side. Inhale. (Photo No. 90).

PICTURE 90

Golden cock stands on one leg

(RIGHT)

Take a small step to the rear with your right foot and take your right palm down to your right side, then bring your left knee and palm upward so that your left elbow is now on your left knee. Exhale as you step down and in as you lift your knee. This is the same group of movements as before in the second third. Bring your right palm upward so that it is near your left elbow and turn both palms up. Still part of that last in-breath. (Photo No.91). Take your right palm back to your rear, the N.E. corner, and as you step to the rear with your left foot. Now do three **Repulse monkey** moves (Photos No. 34, 35, 36). Repeat (Photo No. 37). Then reapeat **Lift hands.**
In fact we now continue as for the second third up to `high pat on horse'.
Repeat Photos 16-21, and then Photos 38 and 39.

PICTURE 91

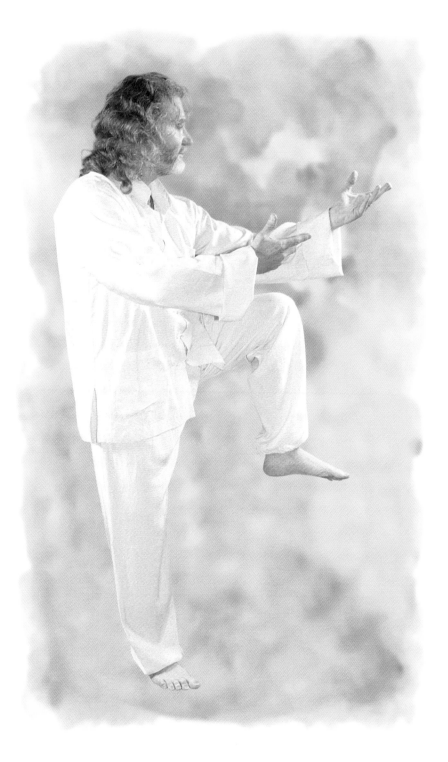

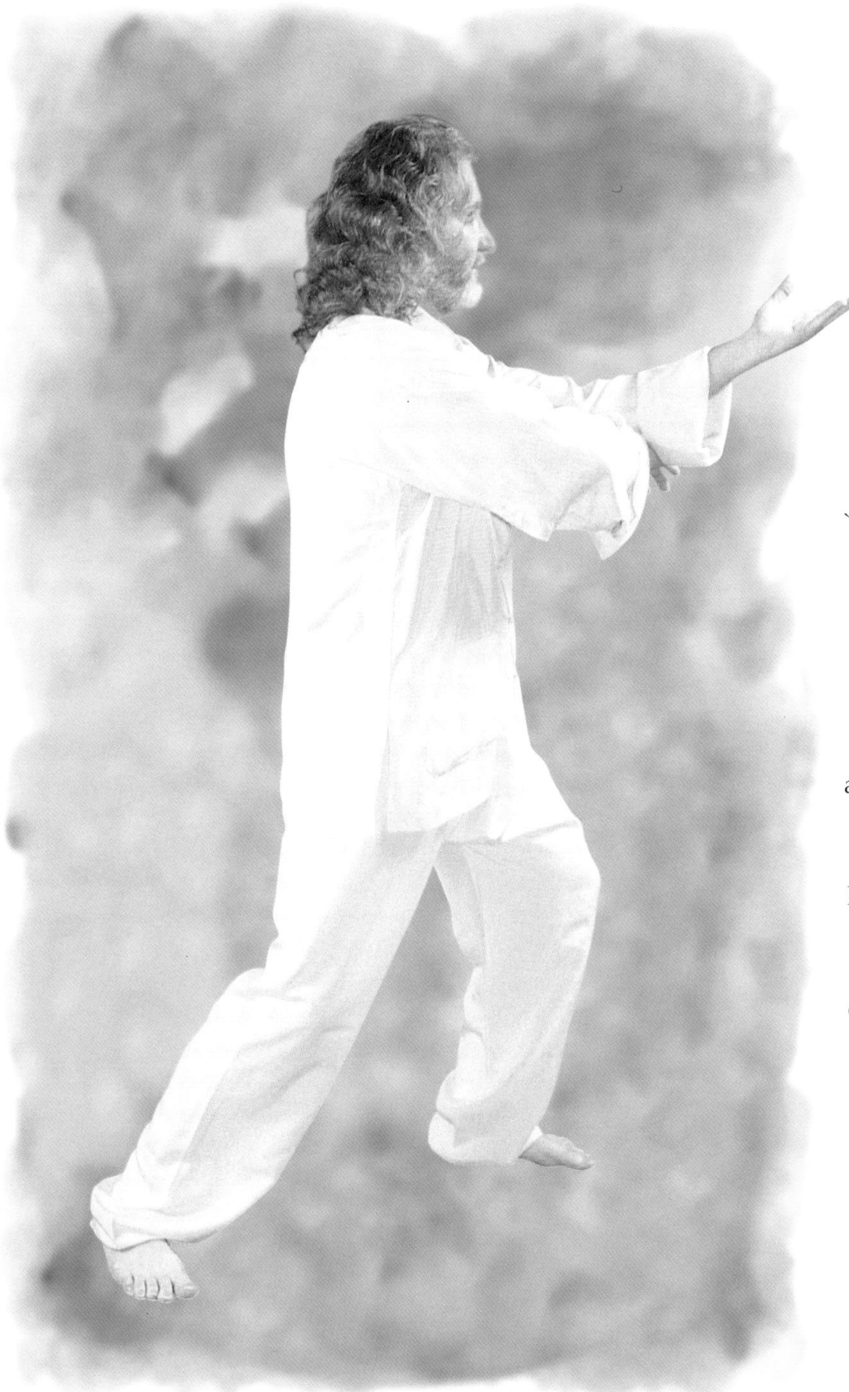

White snake puts out tongue

From **'fan through back'** the posture called **'turn around and chop with fist'** is now called **'white snake puts out tongue'**. It is the same as in Photo No. 40 only the fist is not held. Instead, use an open palm. Keep going as in the second third, Photos 25, 26 up to `punch'. Now repeat: Photo No. 41. **Grasping swallow's tail** is now repeated exactly as in the second third, up to **'single whip'**: photos 7 (slightly different step to begin with) 8, 9, 10, 11, 12, 13, 14 and15. You are now facing the West. Repeat Photos 42, 43, 44, 45, 46. Then Photo No.15.Then you repeat Photos 47and 48. **Inspection of horse's mouth.** From **'high pat on horse'**, step to your left diagonally to gain a bow stance to the west. Inhale. As you transfer your weight onto your left foot, slide your left palm over your right wrist right up to your elbow and exhale. (Photo No. 92).

PICTURE 92

Cross over and kick with right heel

A weighted turn. The left toes turn to the North as your left palm wards off overhead and your right palm guards under your left axilla. Inhale. Open both palms as for a kick and kick with your right heel to the East. (Photo No. 93). Inhale as you cross your arms and exhale as your palms go out, then inhale as you kick.

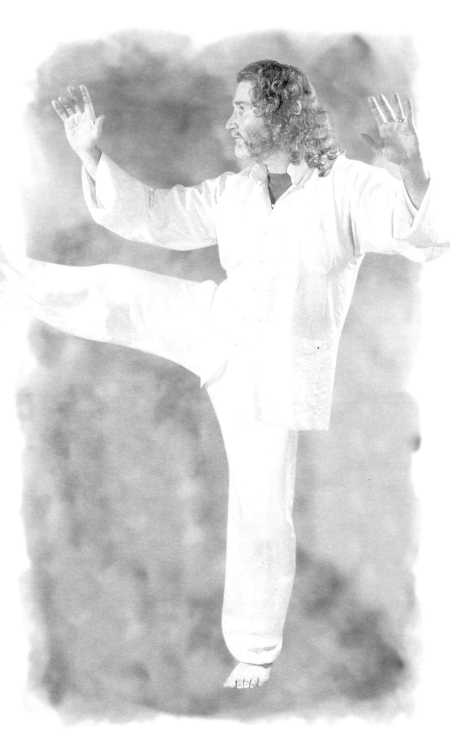

PICTURE 93

Punch to groin

From the last posture and with the right knee still held up, place your right fist onto the outside of your right knee as in the second third. Take a step with your right foot forwards so that your toes are pointing to the S.E.. with your right fist still on your right knee. Your left palm is holding the ball over the right knee. Now, as before, take a step to the East with your left foot and as you do this, brush your left knee with your left palm and punch downwards to the area of the groin, a little higher than before. (Photo No. 94). Exhale.

Diagonal P'eng

This is the same posture as in the second third. From the last posture, cross your left wrist under your right forearm and slide your left palm under your right wrist to end up in a p'eng posture into the N.E. as in (Photo No. 41).

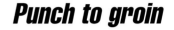
PICTURE 94

Grasping swallow's tail

Exactly as before in the posture of the same name.
Repeat photos 7, (slightly different step) 8, 9, 10, 11, 12, 13, 14 and finish at 'single whip' to the West.

Snake creeps down

This posture ends up in the same position as before but getting into it is a little different. As you shuffle backwards, bring your right palm down in an arc to just in front of your left palm. (Photo No. 95)

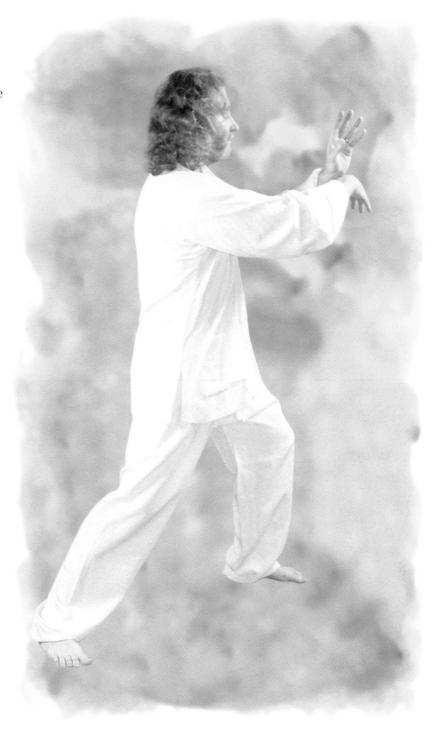

PICTURE **95**

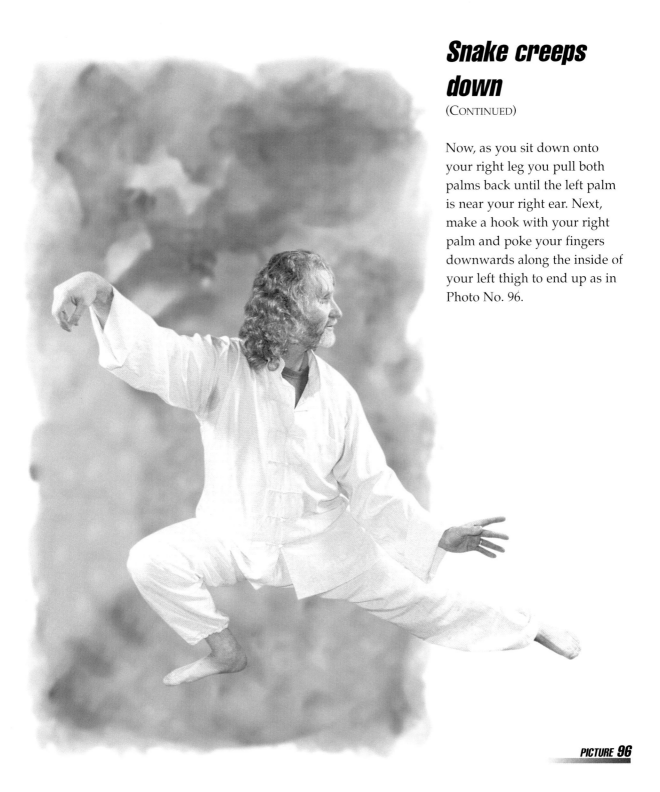

Snake creeps down

(CONTINUED)

Now, as you sit down onto your right leg you pull both palms back until the left palm is near your right ear. Next, make a hook with your right palm and poke your fingers downwards along the inside of your left thigh to end up as in Photo No. 96.

PICTURE 96

Step forward to seven stars

Come back up in the same way as before, but this time as you bring your right foot up, place the toes down in front in a toe stance to the West as you cross your wrists in front holding two fists. (Photo No. 97). Exhale.

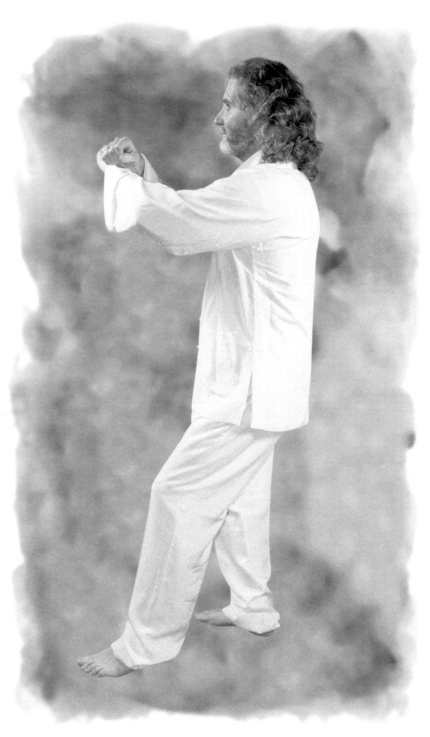

PICTURE 97

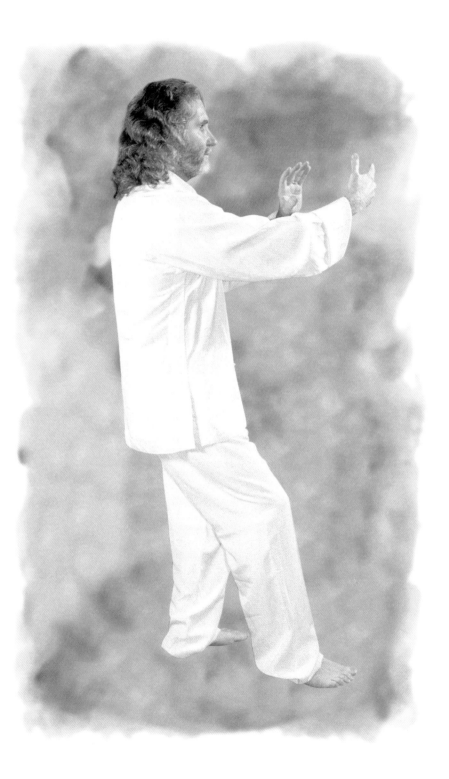

Ride tiger back to mountain

From the last posture, open both palms as if holding a small ball and start to take a right step backwards. (Photo No. 98).

PICTURE **98**

Ride tiger back to mountain

(Continued)

Inhale as you hold this ball, and out as you enter the next posture. Place your right foot down, and as you sit back onto it, open both palms to a sort of 'stork spreads wings' posture. Exhale. (Photo No. 99).

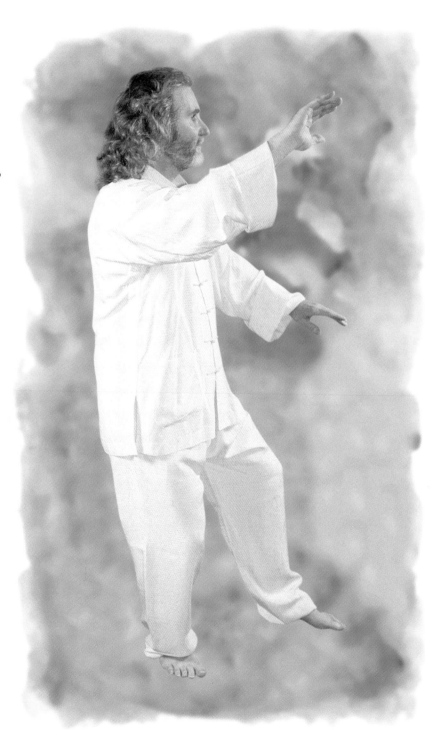

PICTURE **99**

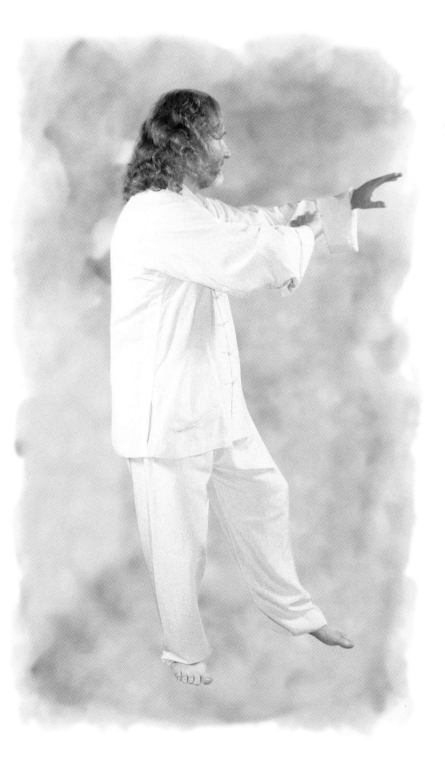

Spin around and lotus kick

Bring your left palm up and
your right palm down to meet
as shown with the left on
the outside. Inhale.
(Photo No. 100).

Spin around and lotus kick

(Continued)

Turn your shoulders slightly to your left and as you spin right around on the ball of your right foot, your right palm is pushed out so that you end up in the exact opposite position you started from. The left foot is to the rear and the weight is now placed on it. (Photo No. 101).

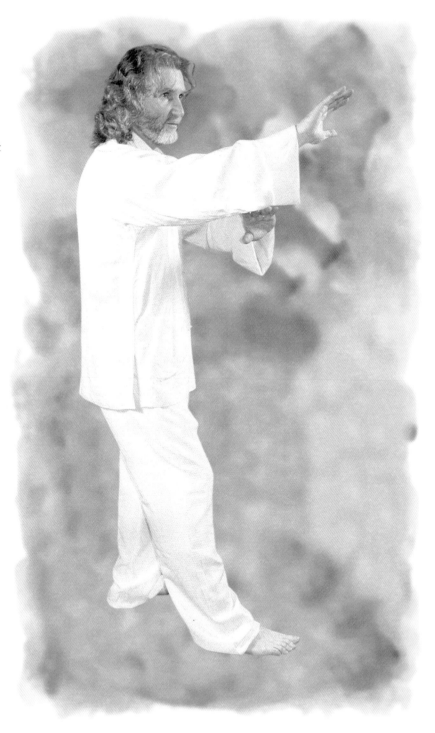

PICTURE 101

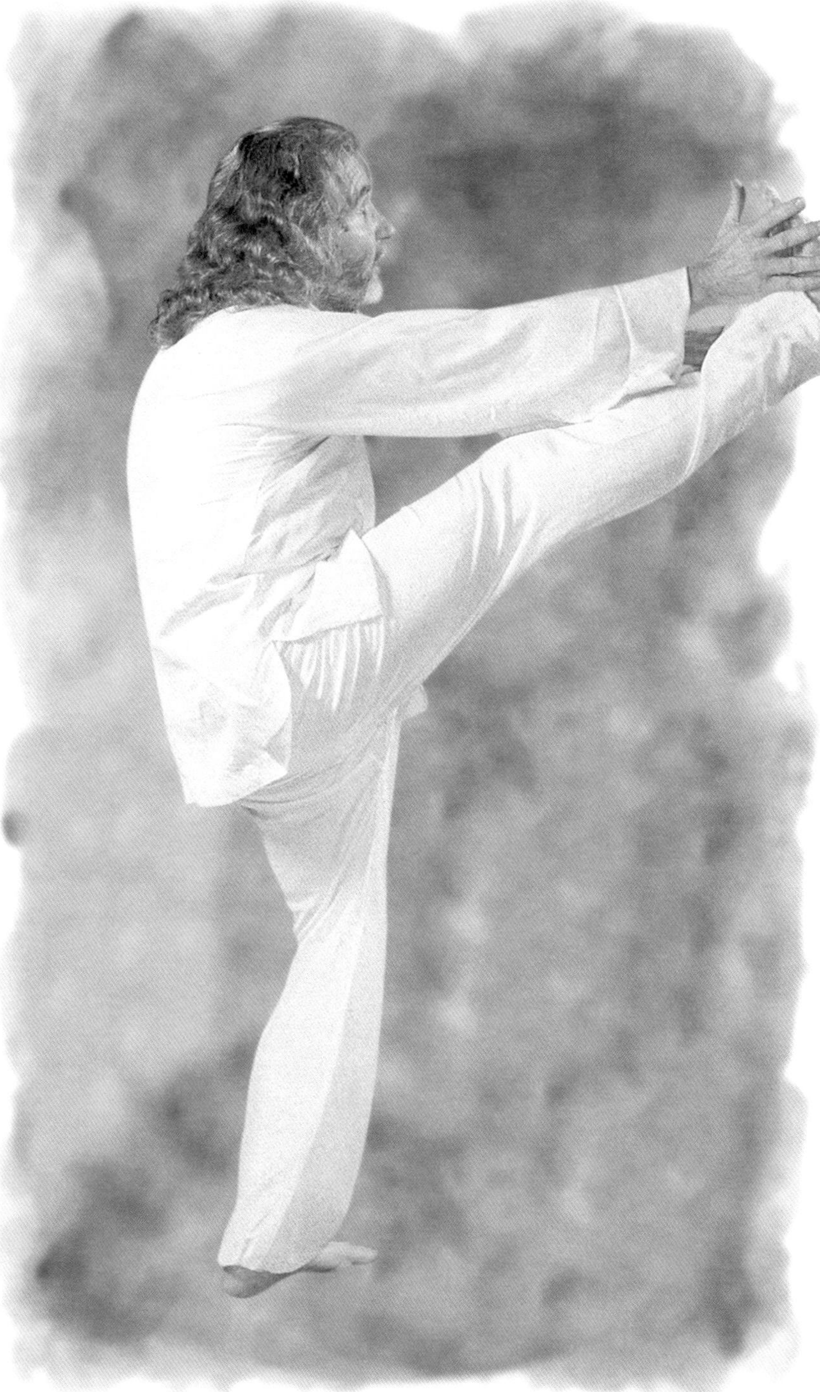

Spin around and lotus kick

(CONTINUED)

Take your palms into the N.W corner by turning your waist. Bring your right foot up in an arc from left over to the right as both palms strike the right foot as shown. The palms are travelling to the left while the foot is travelling to your right. (Photo No. 102).

PICTURE **102**

Spin around and lotus kick

(CONTINUED)

Your right foot ends up into the N.W. corner with toes facing to the N.W. Your palms continue the counter clockwise circle to end up over your right knee. (Photo No. 103). Inhale as you kick, and out for the next posture.

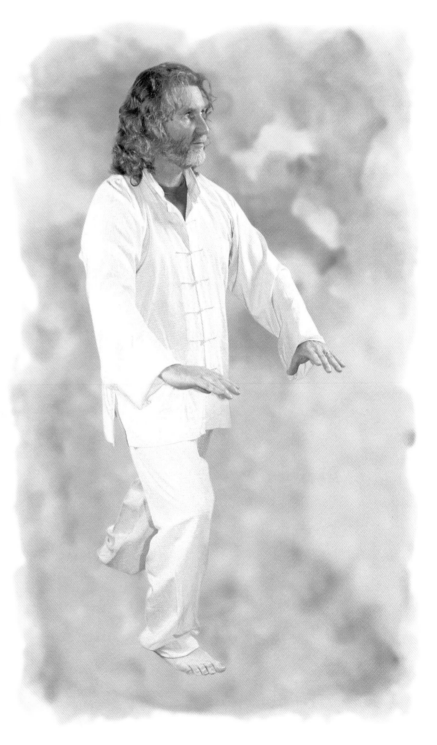

PICTURE **103**

Phoenix punch

Lift both palms up so that they form two fists facing each other. (Photo No. 104).

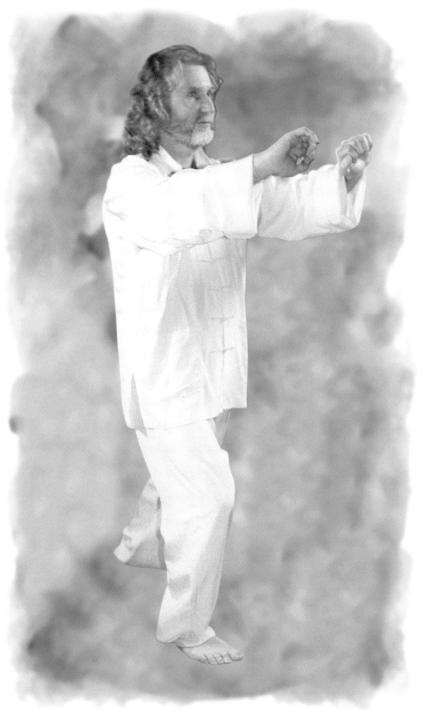

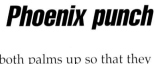

PICTURE *104*

Shoot tiger

Turn your hips slightly to your right as your left fist strikes downwards and your right fist moves over your head. This is also part of your last out breath. (Photo No. 105).

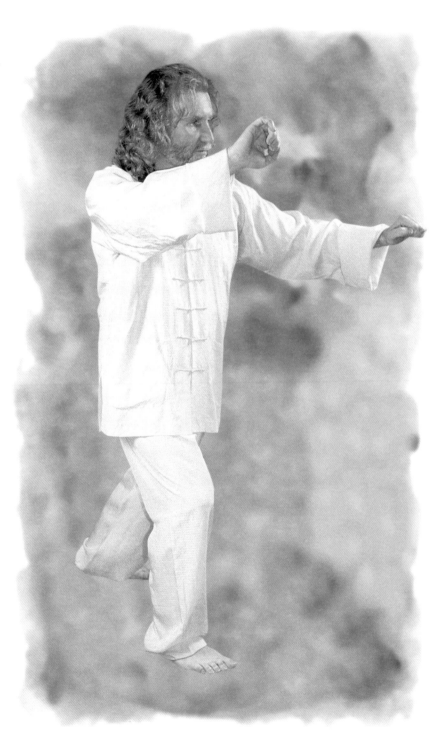

PICTURE 105

Step up, parry and punch

Finish off exactly the same way as for the first and second thirds. Turn your left palm over as you turn your left foot back to the S.W. Your right fist follows your left palm as it rises in an arc to your left ear while your right foot lifts up. (Photo No. 106).

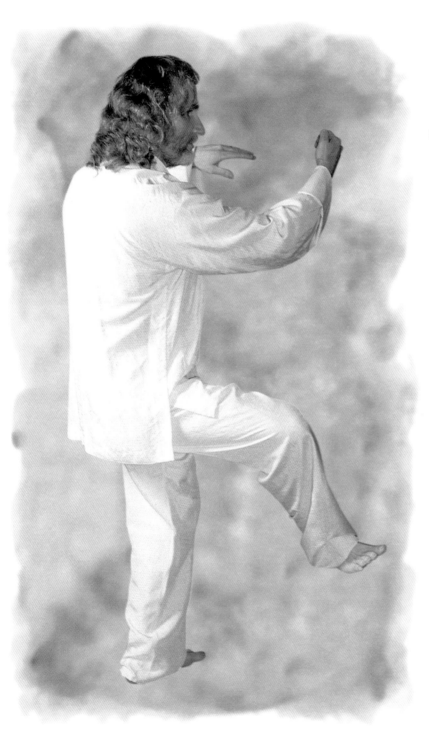

Step up, parry and punch

(Continued)

Now as before step down with your right foot, block and strike to the West with your left palm as in Photo No. 107.

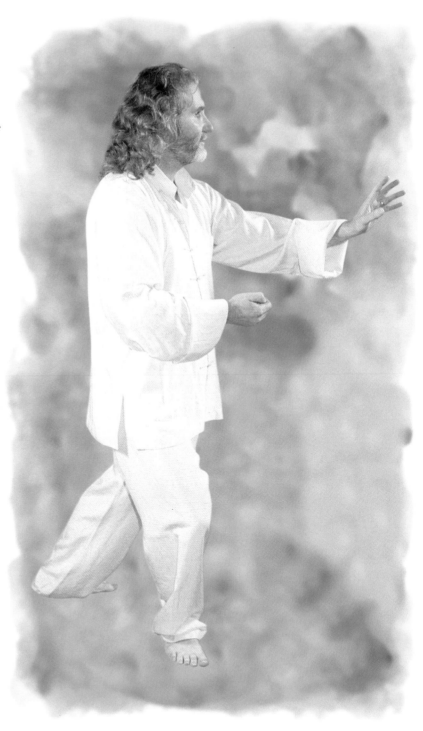

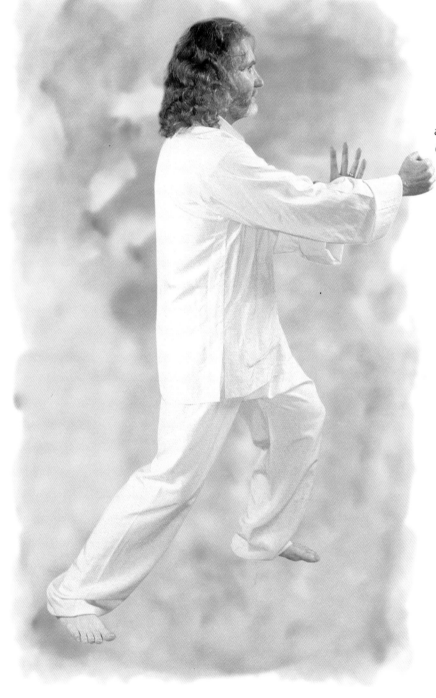

Step up, parry and punch
(CONTINUED)

Step through as in Photo No. 108 and punch. Sit back and push forward exactly the same as in the first and second thirds (Photos 27 & 28). Now perform 'apparent close up' as before. (Photo No. 47).

PICTURE 108

Step up, parry and punch

(CONTINUED)

You have now finished up with your weight on your right leg and arms crossed over your chest. (Photo No. 109).

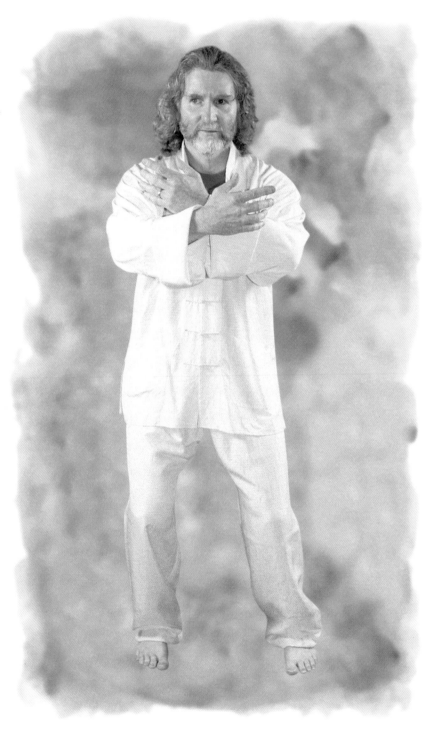

PICTURE 109

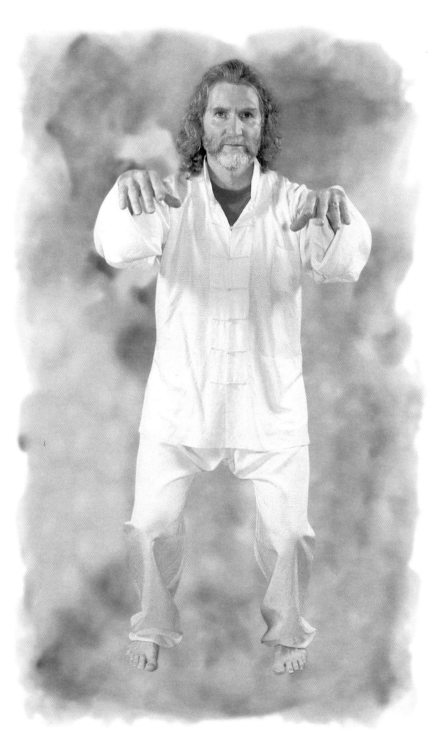

Step up, parry and punch

(CONTINUED)

Lower both palms to your lower abdomen as you make your weight even. As you raise your palms to shoulder height inhale and lower your weight as low as you can go, still keeping your back vertical. (Photo No. 110).

That is the end of the last third, and the end of the Long Form.

PICTURE 110

About the author

ERLE MONTAIGUE has been practising the martial/healing art of T'ai Chi Ch'uan since 1968. His teachers include Master Wong Eog, Master Chu King Hung, and Grand-master Chang Yiu-Chun, one of only two disciples of Yang Shou-hou. Erle became the first student of Master Chu in London in 1973. Chu was one of three disciples of Yang Sau-chung, (1909-1985) the eldest son of the great master Yang Cheng-Fu. Erle was formally introduced to Yang Sau-chung in 1981 when he visited him at his home in Hong-Kong to have his form corrected.

In 1985, Erle and eight of his students became the first Westerners to be asked to perform at the all China National Wushu Tournament in Yinchuan, China. There, Erle was tested by four of the world's greatest Chinese masters and was awarded the degree of "MASTER", the only Westerner to be given this honour. Erle now regards Chang Yiu-Chun as his main teacher from whom he learnt the "Old Yang Style" & The Dim-Mak. Erle's books, videos and articles have helped to change the way that people look at the internal martial arts. His videos are viewed all around the world and his books are sold globally, including China. He is the Chairman of the WORLD TAIJI BOXING ASSOCIATION, Chairman of the WORLD THERAPEUTIC MOVEMENT ASSOCIATION, Vice-Chairman of the FEDERATION OF AUSTRALASIAN WUSHU AND KUNG-FU ORGANIZATIONS, Editor of COMBAT AND HEALING MAGAZINE and has his own column in "Australasian Fighting Arts Magazine." He is also the Australasian Correspondent for Fighting Arts International, the prestigious British International Martial Arts Magazine and writes his own column for this magazine.

In May 1995, Erle Montaigue became the first westerner to go to China to learn from the Original Wudang Shan group, namely one Liang Shiah-kan, the keeper of the original Dim-Mak Qi Disruptive Forms.

For further information on Taijiquan, Qigong, Dim-Mak and Baguazhang, and a catalogue of the author's 190 video titles covering all aspects of these arts, visit the Tai Chi World website at: **http://taichiworld.com**
You can also write to Moon Ta-gu Books, PO Box 792, Murwillumbah NSW 2484, Australia, or email to: **taiji@moontagu.com**

The publishers would like to thank the following sources for their kind permission to reproduce the pictures in this book:
The Image Bank/Tom Owen Edwards 7, Guang Jui Xie 12
Panos Pictures/Jon Spaull 11, Chris Stowers 14
Panos Pictures/Wang Gang Feng 8

Every effort has been made to acknowledge correctly and contact the source and/copyright holder of each picture, and Carlton Books Limited apologises for any unintentional errors or omissions which will be corrected in future editions of this book.